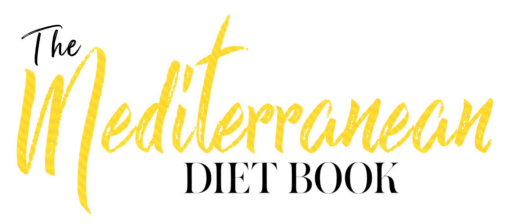

The Mediterranean
DIET BOOK

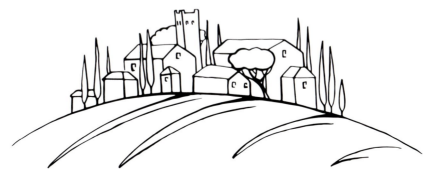

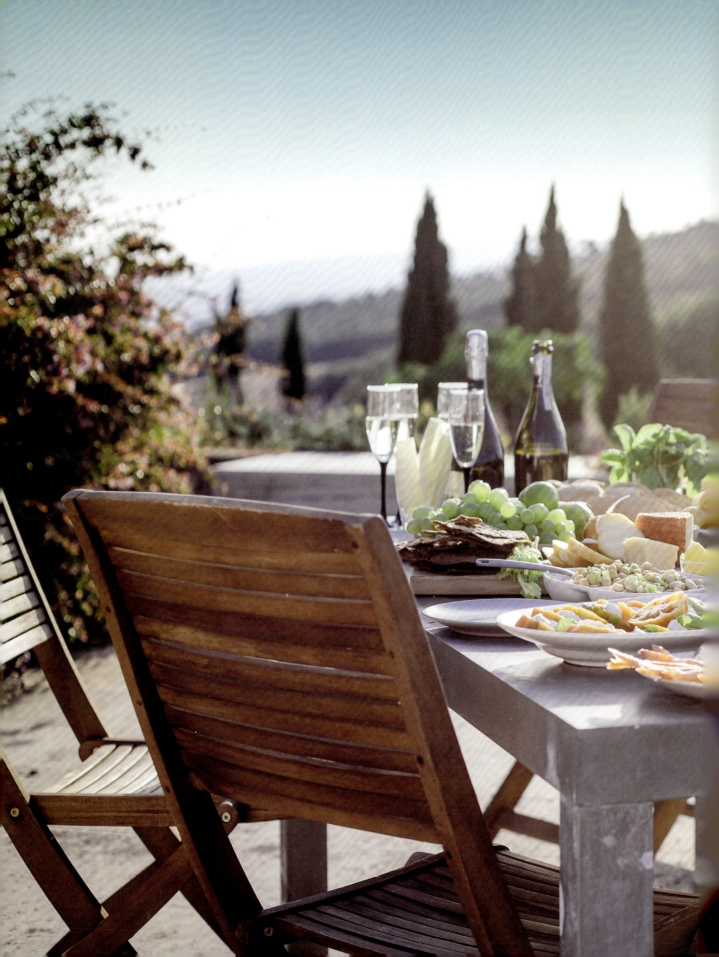

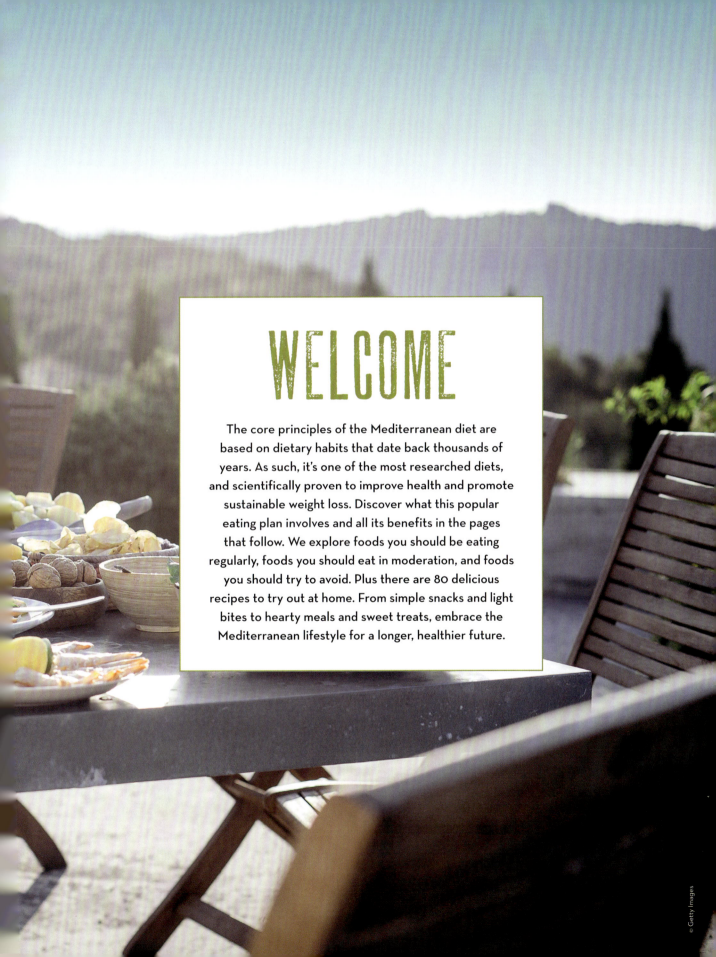

WELCOME

The core principles of the Mediterranean diet are based on dietary habits that date back thousands of years. As such, it's one of the most researched diets, and scientifically proven to improve health and promote sustainable weight loss. Discover what this popular eating plan involves and all its benefits in the pages that follow. We explore foods you should be eating regularly, foods you should eat in moderation, and foods you should try to avoid. Plus there are 80 delicious recipes to try out at home. From simple snacks and light bites to hearty meals and sweet treats, embrace the Mediterranean lifestyle for a longer, healthier future.

CONTENTS

INTRODUCTION

- The origins of the Mediterranean diet 12
- What is the Mediterranean diet? 14
- Benefits of a Mediterranean diet 16
- What to eat & drink 22
- What to have in moderation 24
- What to avoid 25
- The Mediterranean lifestyle 26

LIGHT BITES

- Quilted olive and halloumi loaf 33
- Mediterranean stuffed pepper 35
- Watermelon, mint and feta salad 37
- Ham and manchego croquettes 39
- Sicilian caponata salad 41
- Veggie frittata with Padrón peppers and greens 43
- Tomato bread with anchovies 45
- Gambas with aioli 47
- Fig and goat's cheese puffs 49
- Mediterranean layered sandwiches 51
- Roasted Med veg and feta 53
- Spanish chicken skewers with patatas bravas 55
- Arty pepper focaccia 57
- Mediterranean gratin 59
- Watermelon 'pizza' with feta 61
- Squid salad with garlic and chilli 63
- Spanakopita 65
- Hummus 67
- Tabbouleh 69
- Spanish omelette with saffron aioli 71
- Burrata, bresaola and clementine salad 73
- Baked feta Greek salad with figs 75
- Roasted pepper and garlic bruschetta 77
- Lamb arancini 79
- Halloumi with a chilli kick 81
- Baked stuffed tomatoes with harissa rice 83
- Lamb pitta bites 85
- Baba ganoush 87
- Pissaladière 89
- Polenta bread with antipasti 91

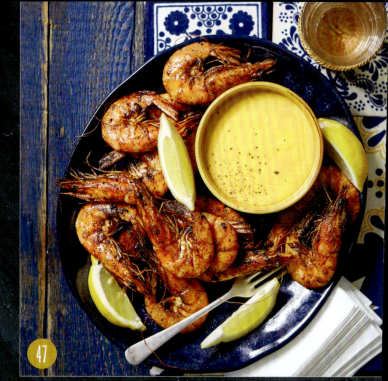

47

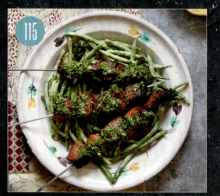

115

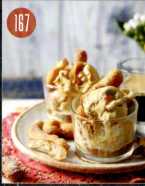

167

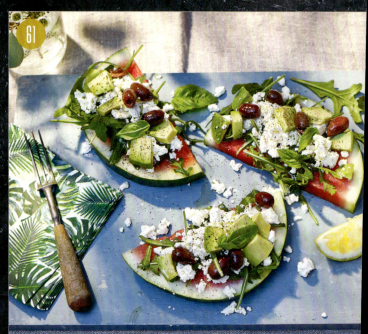

61

MAIN MEALS

Spanish chicken bake 95
White bean & tomato salad 97
Stuffed mackerel 99
Moussaka 101
Mediterranean lamb with feta stuffing 103
Summer ratatouille 105
Chicken stuffed with basil 107
Timballo Siciliano 109
Fisherman's sea bream with aioli 111
Vegetarian lasagne 113
Portuguese-style beef skewers with French beans ... 115
Tomato and couscous salad 117
Provençal fish traybake 119
Mediterranean vegetable calzone 121
Lamb cutlets with pea and mint purée 123
Mediterranean veg rolls 125
Catalan fish stew 127
Risotto al funghi 129
Salmon & spaghetti Bolognese 131
Couscous and chickpea salad 133
Paella 135
Mediterranean sea bass bake 137
Mussels with chorizo 139
Med-style chicken with basil and olives 141
Chicken shawarma 143
Greek roast chicken gyros 145
Chicken parmigiana 147
Veal steak with polenta 149
Pork chops with orzo 151
Pork Milanese with saffron risotto 153
Salmon parcels 155
Portuguese sardines 157
Fried squid 159
Falafel halloumi skewers 161

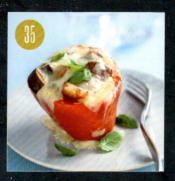
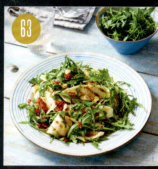
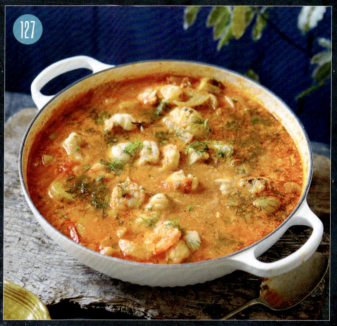
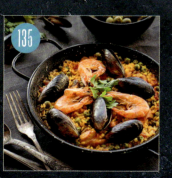
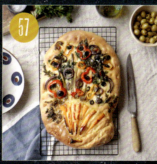

DESSERTS

Tarta di Santiago 165
Churros with salted caramel affogato 167
Gelo di melone 169
Crostata di pistachio con ricotta e limone tart 171
Pasteis de nata 173
Tiramisu 175
Kremsnita 177
Pistachio baklava 179
Crème brûleé 181
Lemon sorbet 183
Crème caramel 185
Basque-style cheesecake with honey roasted figs ... 187
Latte panna cotta 189
Poached pears with ricotta, honey and pine nuts 191
Pistachio, rose and olive oil cake 193
Orange polenta cake 195

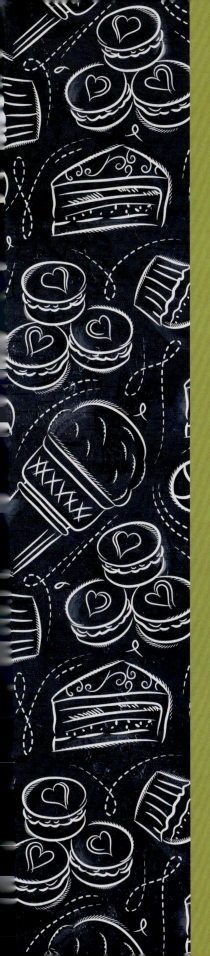
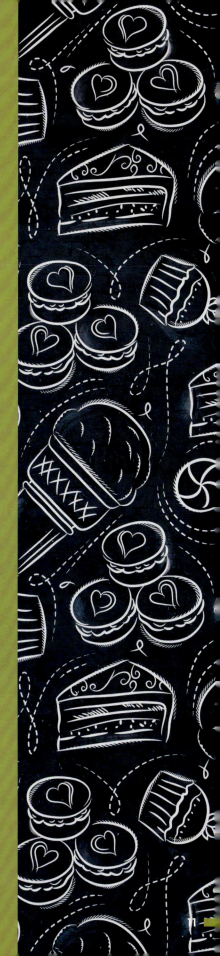

INTRODUCTION

The origins of the Mediterranean diet 12
What is the Mediterranean diet? 14
Benefits of a Mediterranean diet........................16
What to eat & drink 22
What to have in moderation 24
What to avoid 25
The Mediterranean lifestyle 26

INTRODUCTION

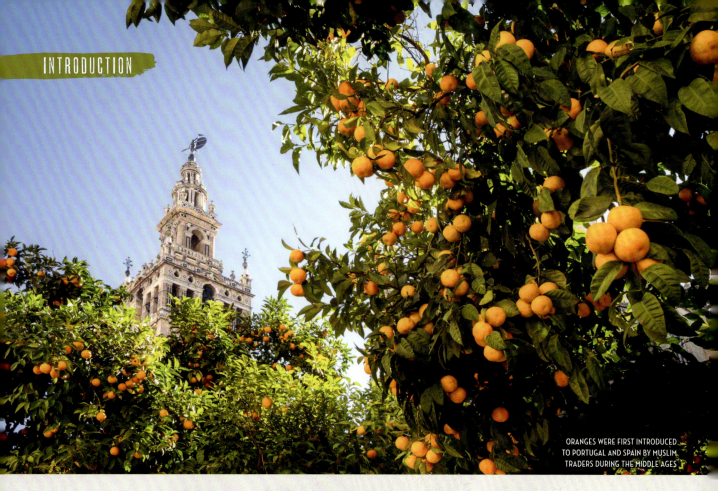

ORANGES WERE FIRST INTRODUCED TO PORTUGAL AND SPAIN BY MUSLIM TRADERS DURING THE MIDDLE AGES

THE ORIGINS OF THE MEDITERRANEAN DIET

AN AUSPICIOUS COMBINATION OF LOCATION, CLIMATE AND HISTORY PROVED TO BE THE RECIPE FOR ONE OF THE WORLD'S HEALTHIEST DIETS

The Mediterranean 'diet' as we know it today has only really been marketed as a specific eating plan over the last few decades, but its core principles are based on dietary habits that date back many thousands of years. The Mediterranean is a unique environment that has nurtured some of the world's most influential civilisations, such as the ancient Egyptians, Greeks and Romans. The cuisines that developed across this region are diverse, but they have all been shaped by their shared geography, climate, staple crops, and millennia of trade and cultural exchange. Broadly speaking, these countries' traditional cuisines are mostly plant-based, with plenty of fresh fruit, vegetables, legumes and cereals, with occasional fish, seafood and dairy, but limited amounts of meat and sweet treats.

Most of the region enjoys a Mediterranean climate, characterised by hot, dry summers and mild, wet winters. There are three key crops that thrive in these conditions: olives, grapes and wheat. Together these are known as the 'Mediterranean triad', and they feature heavily in most of the region's cuisines in the form of olive oil, wine and bread. Ancient civilisations developed agricultural methods to help cultivate their staple crops, such as tiered terraces, to protect against soil erosion on the Mediterranean's many hillsides and mountainsides, and irrigation systems to supply water to the more arid areas. In addition, technological advancements led to inventions like grain mills and olive presses. These made production of otherwise labour-intensive commodities like flour and olive oil far more efficient, and enabled them to be produced in greater quantities.

Mediterranean cuisine has been heavily influenced by occupying powers and trade

THE SEVEN COUNTRIES STUDY

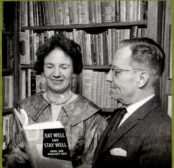

ANCEL KEYS AND HIS WIFE MARGARET CO-WROTE SEVERAL BESTSELLING BOOKS PROMOTING THE BENEFITS OF A MEDITERRANEAN DIET

The Mediterranean diet owes a lot of its popularity to the work of Ancel Keys, an American physiologist who investigated the links between diet and heart disease. In 1956, he began the Seven Countries Study, a long-term project examining the relationships between people's diets and lifestyles and their risk of heart disease and stroke. Teams spent years gathering health and lifestyle data from thousands of volunteers in the USA, Japan, Finland, the Netherlands, Italy, Greece, and parts of the former Yugoslavia (now Croatia and Serbia).

The first results were published in the '70s, and Keys' data showed that high blood cholesterol levels were linked to an increased risk of heart disease. He also found that, despite having a fairly high fat intake, Mediterranean volunteers generally had a much lower risk of heart disease compared to American and Northern European participants. Keys hypothesised that the unsaturated fats (such as vegetable oils) that featured heavily in Mediterranean diets had beneficial effects, while the saturated fats in meat and dairy had detrimental effects on heart health. This discovery has been supported by many other scientific studies since, and it played a major role in popularising the Mediterranean-style diet as a means to improve health.

THE MEDITERRANEAN IS A UNIQUE ENVIRONMENT THAT HAS NURTURED SOME OF THE WORLD'S MOST INFLUENTIAL CIVILISATIONS

with the wider world. For centuries the Romans dominated the region. Internal trade between the Roman provinces helped to spread regional produce and new imports around the empire, while external trade with India brought exotic spices to the region. Following the Islamic conquest of the Iberian Peninsula and Sicily in the Middle Ages, Muslim traders introduced various ingredients and crops from the Middle East and beyond, including apricots, aubergines (eggplant), carrots, citrus fruits, rice and sugarcane. Further significant imports came in the 16th century following Spanish expeditions to the New World. Explorers returned with several popular additions, including potatoes, peppers and tomatoes. Today, it is almost impossible to imagine Mediterranean food without the latter.

While trade did spread common crops and produce throughout the Mediterranean, each region retained its own distinctive cuisines, cooking techniques and preferred ingredients. Take a simple dish like a stew, and you'll find herby French bouillabaisse, hearty Italian ragu, warming Turkish güveçs, fragrantly spiced Moroccan tagines, and many more besides. Even a staple food like bread varies, with the same basic ingredients transformed into regional specialties, such as the baguette, ciabatta, pita, matzo, and khobz. While the modern diet uses the broad, catch-all term of 'Mediterranean', the abundance of regional specialties provide a great deal of variety and inspiration.

The Mediterranean diet itself is a relatively recent concept. The idea of 'Mediterranean' being a cuisine in its own right was popularised by the English food writer Elizabeth David in her hugely influential cookbook, *A Book of Mediterranean Food*, published in 1950. The book was credited with changing English eating habits by reintroducing fresh, colourful recipes to a post-war nation that was weary of rationing. It wasn't until the 1970s, when results from the Seven Countries Study were published (see boxout), that the scientific community and the general public began to take notice of the Mediterranean diet. In the decades since, there have been thousands of studies into Mediterranean-style diets, corroborating many of those initial findings and uncovering even more fantastic health benefits. It should come as no surprise, then, that the Mediterranean diet is one of the most widely followed eating plans in the world today, and has remained consistently popular while countless fad diets have come and gone.

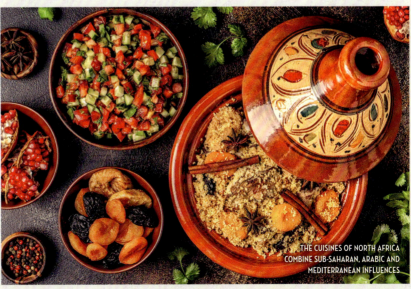

THE CUISINES OF NORTH AFRICA COMBINE SUB-SAHARAN, ARABIC AND MEDITERRANEAN INFLUENCES

INTRODUCTION

WHAT IS THE MEDITERRANEAN DIET?

THIS POPULAR EATING PLAN HAS BEEN SCIENTIFICALLY PROVEN TO IMPROVE YOUR HEALTH AND PROMOTE SUSTAINABLE WEIGHT LOSS, BUT WHAT DOES A MEDITERRANEAN DIET INVOLVE?

Starting any new diet can be an intimidating process. You may be faced with an overwhelming amount of information about all the foods you can and can't eat, or you might even be forced to restock your cupboards with a strange selection of expensive and unfamiliar new ingredients. Thankfully, this is not the case here! The Mediterranean diet was inspired by the traditional eating habits of people from that part of the world (specifically parts of Italy, Greece and what is now Croatia). Although globalisation means that many Mediterraneans today have adopted more 'Western' eating habits, the diet itself is based on research conducted between the 1950s and 1970s when people ate less meat and fewer convenience foods. Eating the Mediterranean way is incredibly simple, and doesn't rely on any obscure, hard-to-find ingredients. The focus is on fresh, unrefined produce that you can find in any greengrocer's or supermarket.

In general, the diet consists mainly of wholegrain products such as bread, pasta and rice, plus plenty of fresh fruits, vegetables, legumes, nuts and seeds. These should make up most of your daily intake. Olive oil is used liberally for cooking, baking and in dressings, replacing the butter or lard often used in other cuisines. Antioxidant-packed red wine is also enjoyed in moderation, typically one or two glasses with meals a few times a week. Fish, seafood, poultry and eggs are typically eaten a few times a week, while full-fat dairy

THERE IS NO CALORIE COUNTING INVOLVED, AND NO FOODS ARE EXPRESSLY FORBIDDEN

TIP
If reducing your meat intake is daunting, try making the change gradually over a few months.

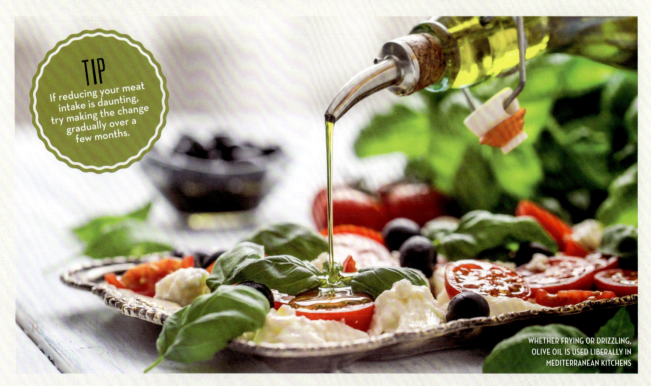

WHETHER FRYING OR DRIZZLING, OLIVE OIL IS USED LIBERALLY IN MEDITERRANEAN KITCHENS

products like cheese and yoghurt feature in modest daily amounts. Red meat is eaten less often, or in much smaller portions, than in the standard Western diet, and sweet treats like cakes and pastries are enjoyed as treats a few times a month.

A key principle of the diet is quality over quantity. For example, by choosing wholegrain or wholewheat products over refined 'white' versions, you are getting more beneficial fibre; full-fat dairy products are more filling and satisfying than processed low-fat options; and reducing your meat intake may mean you can afford to choose higher-quality, higher-welfare and/or organic cuts. Where possible, try to buy local, seasonal produce too. Not only will this help to ensure your diet contains a wide variety of vitamins and minerals, but you'll get to enjoy fruits and vegetables when they are at their best. There's no contest between a fragrant, sweet strawberry that's in season compared to a bland, watery, out-of-season import.

The Mediterranean diet is nowhere near as restrictive as other diets. There is no calorie counting involved, and no foods are expressly forbidden, so you can still have the occasional treat. *Occasional* is the key word here, though. A juicy steak or a slice of cake should be enjoyed a couple of times a month, rather than daily or weekly. While the diet doesn't have strict rules, it's best not to stray too far from the core principles. The diet is based on the traditional eating habits of the region, where people would make meals from scratch using fresh produce. As common sense would tell you, ordering a takeaway pizza for dinner every day would not be a particularly good interpretation of a Mediterranean diet!

It's important to note that the Mediterranean diet is not a crash diet. It is a long-term lifestyle change that promotes steady, sustainable weight loss (when combined with reasonable portion control), or makes it easy to maintain a healthy weight, depending on your needs. A common problem for crash dieters is that, after they stop dieting, they end up regaining some, if not all of the weight they initially lost. By adopting healthy eating habits that are easy to stick to, you will be far more likely to keep weight off for good. The Mediterranean diet should ideally be something you choose to continue for the rest of your life in order to enjoy its wide-ranging health benefits.

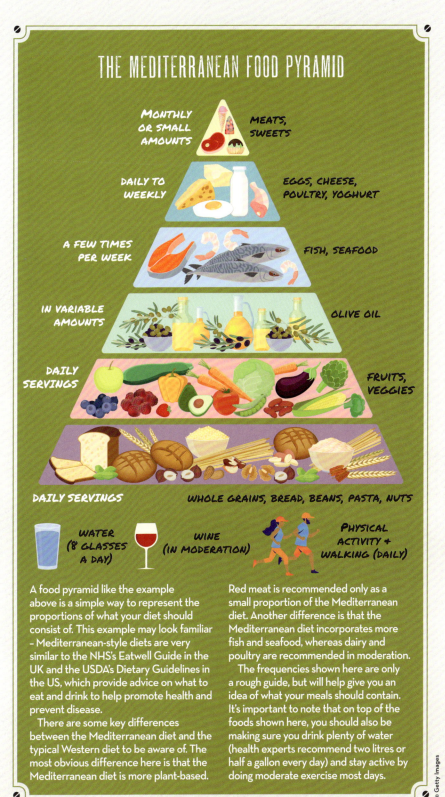

A food pyramid like the example above is a simple way to represent the proportions of what your diet should consist of. This example may look familiar – Mediterranean-style diets are very similar to the NHS's Eatwell Guide in the UK and the USDA's Dietary Guidelines in the US, which provide advice on what to eat and drink to help promote health and prevent disease.

There are some key differences between the Mediterranean diet and the typical Western diet to be aware of. The most obvious difference here is that the Mediterranean diet is more plant-based. Red meat is recommended only as a small proportion of the Mediterranean diet. Another difference is that the Mediterranean diet incorporates more fish and seafood, whereas dairy and poultry are recommended in moderation.

The frequencies shown here are only a rough guide, but will help give you an idea of what your meals should contain. It's important to note that on top of the foods shown here, you should also be making sure you drink plenty of water (health experts recommend two litres or half a gallon every day) and stay active by doing moderate exercise most days.

INTRODUCTION

BENEFITS OF A MEDITERRANEAN DIET

FIND OUT WHY SWITCHING TO A MEDITERRANEAN DIET COULD BE THE BEST INVESTMENT YOU EVER MAKE IN YOUR HEALTH

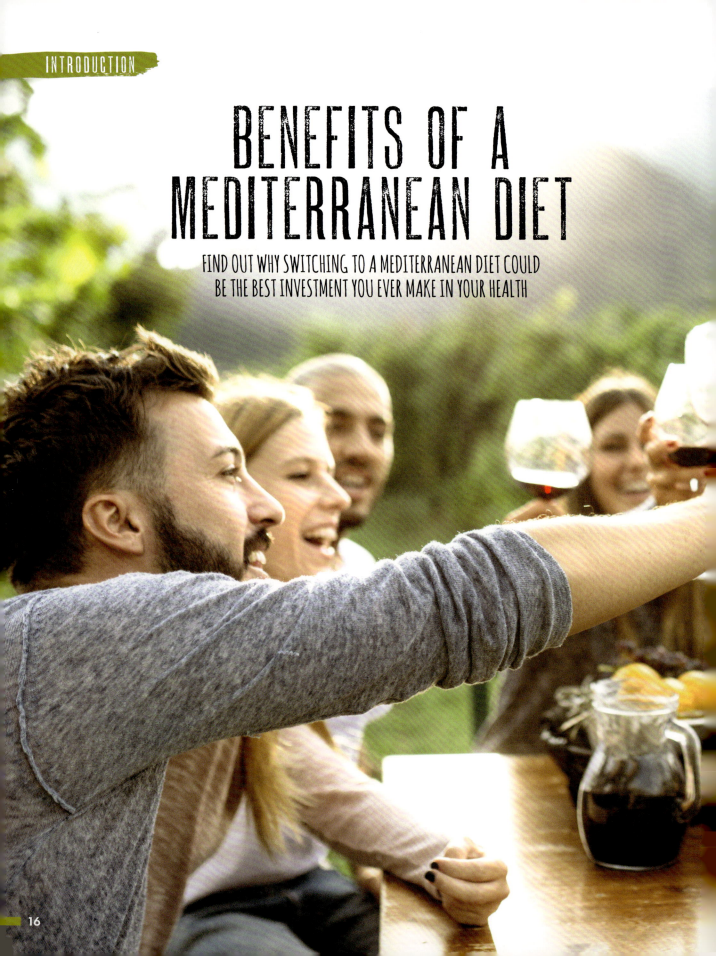

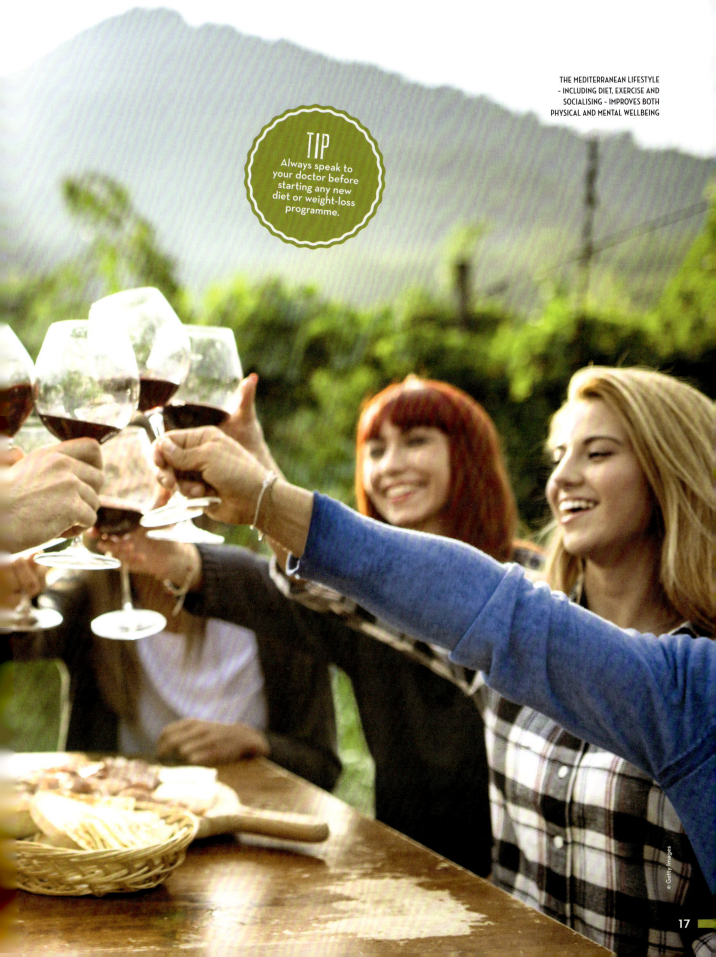

INTRODUCTION

There are plenty of diets out there that boast seemingly miraculous results, but very few are supported by decades of rigorous scientific research and recommended by health professionals. Mediterranean-style diets have been the subject of thousands of studies over the years, and scientists continue to learn more about their long-term effects on our health. The Mediterranean diet has been shown time and time again to be one of the healthiest ways to eat, and its benefits extend far beyond the typical diet selling point of weight loss. This lifestyle can have a considerable impact on both your physical and mental wellbeing, and it's even good for the environment, too. Here are just some of the ways a Mediterranean diet can change your life...

REDUCE YOUR RISK OF DISEASE
One of the best-studied aspects of the Mediterranean diet is its link to a lower risk of cardiovascular disease (CVD), such as heart attacks and strokes. CVD is the leading cause of death globally; in many cases, lifestyle factors play a major role in the development of CVD, and typically a diet that's high in saturated fat and sugar increases your risk. The Mediterranean diet is relatively low in saturated fat as it is less reliant on meat and dairy, so it naturally helps to minimise your risk of CVD. One study revealed that a Mediterranean-style diet can cut the risk of developing CVD by 25%, while another found that it reduces the risk of death from stroke by about 30%.

Having high blood cholesterol levels is another major risk factor for developing heart problems or suffering a stroke, but the balance of the *type* of cholesterol in our blood is also important. High levels of LDL (low-density lipoprotein) cholesterol can build up in the blood vessels and lead to blockages, while HDL (high-density lipoprotein) cholesterol is beneficial because it helps to remove LDL from the blood. Replacing saturated fats with unsaturated fats helps to reduce levels of harmful HDL and boosts levels of the beneficial LDL kind.

Besides CVD, the Mediterranean diet can help reduce the risk of other diseases such as type 2 diabetes, arthritis, cancer and dementia. These conditions have all been linked to chronic inflammation, where the body continues to produce an immune response when it doesn't need to. This in turn puts a lot of stress on cells and causes damage. The Mediterranean

> A MEDITERRANEAN-STYLE DIET CAN REDUCE THE RISK OF DEVELOPING CARDIOVASCULAR DISEASE BY **25%** AND DEATH FROM STROKE BY ABOUT **30%**

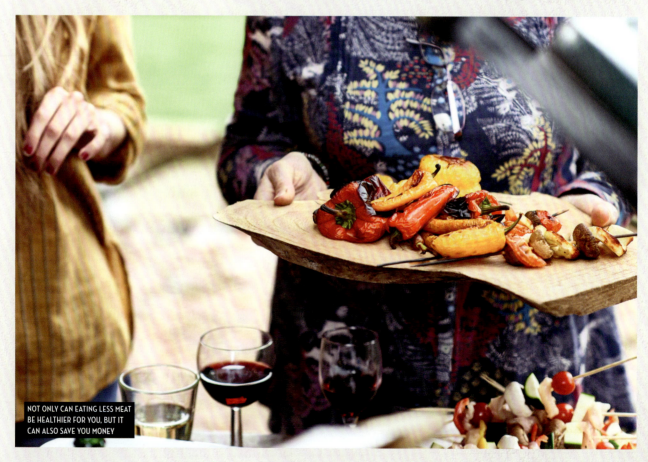

NOT ONLY CAN EATING LESS MEAT BE HEALTHIER FOR YOU, BUT IT CAN ALSO SAVE YOU MONEY

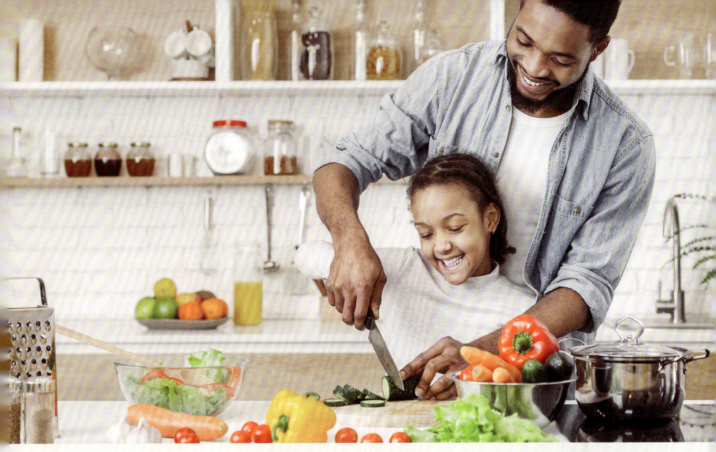

THE EARLIER YOU CAN START FOLLOWING A MEDITERRANEAN-STYLE DIET, THE GREATER ITS BENEFITS WILL BE

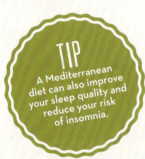

TIP A Mediterranean diet can also improve your sleep quality and reduce your risk of insomnia.

diet has been found to reduce levels of inflammation because it incorporates foods that are rich in polyphenols and antioxidants. These compounds have a protective effect in the body, and have been shown to help reduce and even repair cell damage.

IMPROVE YOUR MENTAL HEALTH

We all have certain comfort foods that make us feel good, but our diet as a whole can have a more profound impact on our mental health. Research has found that a Western-style diet (high in refined grains, sugar and fat) can increase your risk of depression and anxiety. However, Mediterranean-style diets can decrease the risk of depression by 30%, and not just in adults. Mental health is a growing issue among young people, but one study found that adhering to a Mediterranean diet can help to reduce the risk of depression in adolescence.

The diet can also help to protect your overall brain health and cognitive function in later life. One study looked at the dietary habits of people in their 70s and performed brain scans to track changes in their brain volume (which naturally declines in old age). They found that participants who adhered more strictly to a Mediterranean-style diet tended to

WATCHING YOUR WEIGHT

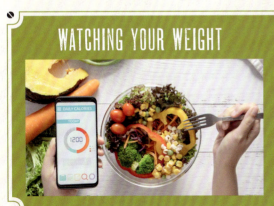

If weight loss is a goal for you, adopting a Mediterranean lifestyle can help you achieve this safely and sustainably. After a few weeks on the diet, many people find that weight loss occurs as a natural consequence, particularly if they have switched from a diet that is high in fat and sugar. If you are already a healthy weight, the Mediterranean diet combined with regular, moderate activity should make this easy to maintain without having to give it much thought. However, the diet does still rely on having reasonable portion sizes, and you might find that the things you are supposed to have 'in moderation' slowly become more regular habits. This may be a struggle at first, so you might want to start a food diary to track exactly what you're eating and how often you are having things like meat, dairy and desserts. It can also be useful to keep an eye on your calorie intake, at least to begin with while you adapt to the new diet – apps like MyFitnessPal make this more convenient.

INTRODUCTION

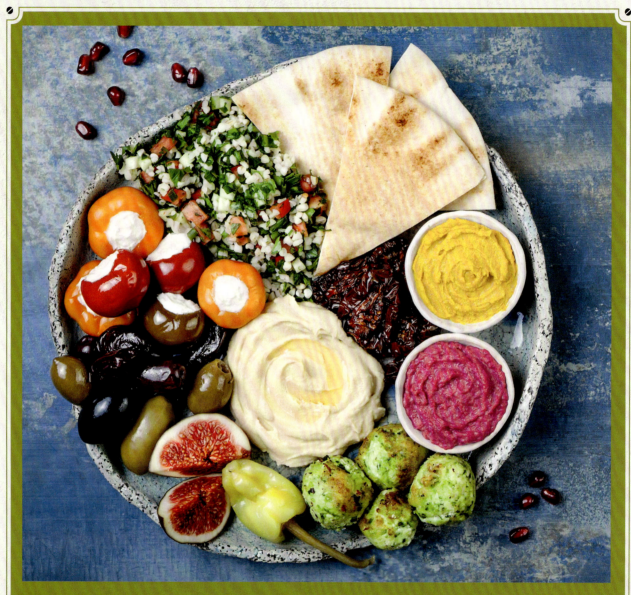

MEAT-FREE MEDITERRANEAN

The Mediterranean diet is naturally less reliant on meat and dairy than a typical Western diet, so it is very simple to adapt for pescatarians, vegetarians and vegans. A lot of Mediterranean dishes are naturally vegetarian or vegan due to the diet being largely plant-based, and its use of olive oil instead of butter. Meat substitutes such as soya or tofu (made from soybeans) can also be included in a Mediterranean diet. However, stick to fresh produce as much as possible, and keep an eye on the ingredients lists for any meat/dairy-free alternative products that you buy. Some items may contain added sugar or salt for extra flavour; nut milks are a common example of this, so look for unsweetened options or try making your own.

If you follow a vegetarian or vegan lifestyle, it is a good idea to speak to your doctor or a qualified nutritionist before adopting a Mediterranean diet. Fish, meat and dairy products contain important nutrients for our bodies that you may struggle to get enough of from other food groups, so you might be advised to take supplements.

> THE EARLIER YOU ADOPT A MEDITERRANEAN DIET, THE GREATER THE LONG-TERM BENEFITS WILL BE, BUT IT'S NEVER TOO LATE TO START

lose less of their total brain volume when compared to others. Other studies have found that a Mediterranean diet can help to protect people's memory and general cognitive abilities as they age.

YOU'LL LIVE LONGER
Researchers from Harvard University found that a Mediterranean diet can even improve longevity. They studied the impact that diet has on telomeres – structures at the end of our chromosomes that protect them from damage. Scientists use telomere length as a marker for aging and life expectancy: in general, shorter telomeres are associated with a reduced life expectancy and a higher risk of developing chronic disease. The more closely people followed a Mediterranean-style diet, the longer their telomeres tended to be, indicating a better life expectancy.

The earlier you adopt a Mediterranean diet, the greater the long-term benefits will be, but it's never too late to start. Studies have found that people who switch to the diet in their fifties and sixties were less likely to experience chronic health problems in later life compared to those with less-healthy diets. Since prevention is better than cure, the Mediterranean diet can be an incredibly effective tool to promote healthy aging and improved quality of life in our later years.

IT CAN SAVE YOU MONEY
The Mediterranean lifestyle emphasises the importance of cooking fresh produce from scratch. While it may not be as convenient as ordering a takeaway or buying a microwave meal, it's certainly better for your health – and your wallet! One study found that participants who switched to a Mediterranean diet over a 34-week period ended up cutting their grocery bills by over 50%! It can be really eye opening to see how much it is possible to save when you reduce your meat intake and take things like ready meals, high-sugar snacks and fizzy drinks out of the equation. The added bonus of spending less on food overall is that you have the option to invest more in quality (such as higher-welfare meat and dairy, and sustainably sourced fish) should you so choose.

IT'S MORE SUSTAINABLE
On the Mediterranean diet we are encouraged to eat local and seasonal produce as much as possible. This can have a dramatic impact on your carbon footprint compared to a typical Western diet. See if there are any farmers' markets near you to make the most of local produce – you might find them cheaper than the supermarkets, too. Diets that take a more plant-based approach have a lower environmental impact than those that rely more heavily on meat and dairy, so it's naturally a greener option. The Mediterranean diet can also be adapted for vegetarians and vegans (see the 'Meat-free Mediterranean' boxout) which can make it even more environmentally friendly.

IT'S EASY TO STICK TO
A major problem with many diets is that they are often intended to be temporary quick fixes, or they are so restrictive that sticking with them in the long-term is simply unrealistic. One reason why the Mediterranean diet is so popular is because it is a common-sense approach – there are no gimmicks, no starving yourself, and no need to cut out entire food groups. Convenience is key for something to be sustainable, and on a Mediterranean diet, all the ingredients you'll need can be found at your regular food stores. What's more, there's such a huge variety of Mediterranean recipes available to try, you won't end up bored from eating the same bland diet meals every day. You don't have to worry about 'ruining' your diet if you have a treat every once in a while either; as long as you take the Mediterranean approach most of the time, you will enjoy the diet's health benefits.

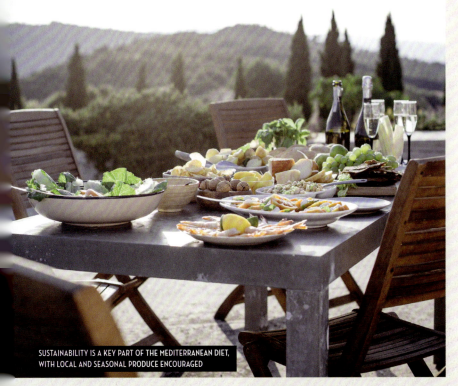
SUSTAINABILITY IS A KEY PART OF THE MEDITERRANEAN DIET, WITH LOCAL AND SEASONAL PRODUCE ENCOURAGED

INTRODUCTION

WHAT TO EAT & DRINK

IN A MEDITERRANEAN DIET, THESE FOODS AND DRINKS WILL MAKE UP THE MAJORITY OF YOUR MEALS AND SHOULD BE ENJOYED EVERY DAY

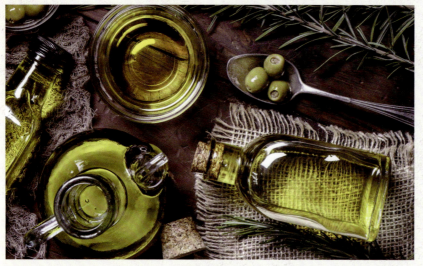

OLIVE OIL

Olive oil is almost synonymous with Mediterranean cuisine. It's the diet's main source of fat, used for frying, roasting, baking and drizzling over salads – whenever you would normally use butter or other types of oil. It's packed with beneficial antioxidants and unsaturated fats, the latter of which have been proven to reduce the risk of heart disease and stroke, compared to the saturated fats in butter. Choose extra-virgin olive oil and buy the best quality for your budget. Avoid varieties that contain a mixture of different oils, or those that come in transparent bottles as sunlight degrades the oil quality.

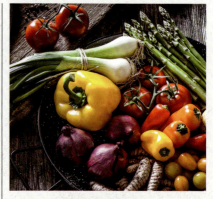

VEGETABLES

Delicious, nutrient-packed vegetables should be a major part of your Mediterranean-style meals, so getting your five (or more) a day should be easy. Each type of vegetable offers a different selection of vitamins and minerals, so aim to eat a variety – from starchy potatoes and earthy beetroot (beets) to crunchy carrots and crisp greens. Fresh, seasonal veg is the best option, but frozen and tinned are better than none. The Mediterranean diet is less reliant on meat, meaning vegetables are often the main event. Although they're not technically veg, mushrooms bring a lovely 'meatiness' to recipes as well.

GRAINS

Cereals such as wheat are among the most important crops in the Mediterranean. The grains from these plants make up a significant portion of the diet, often in the form of bread, pasta and rice. Other grains commonly used around the Mediterranean include barley, oats, durum wheat (for couscous) and corn (for polenta). Use wholegrain varieties where possible – they contain more of the all-important fibre that makes grains so beneficial for digestive health. Diets that include plenty of wholegrain foods are linked to a reduced risk of heart disease, obesity, type 2 diabetes, and even some forms of cancer.

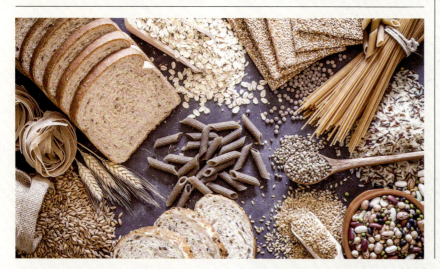

PULSES

Pulses like beans, peas and lentils are important sources of protein, fibre, vitamins and minerals. They make a nutritious addition to meals, as well as providing bulk and texture to stews, soups, salads, dips and more. If you don't already eat a lot of pulses, it is recommended that you increase your intake gradually and drink plenty of water, otherwise the sudden increase in fibre can cause some temporary digestive discomfort. Some plant-based meat alternatives like tofu are made from pulses, but avoid brands that contain highly processed oils, added sugar and excess salt if you are using these.

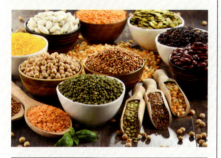

COFFEE AND TEAS

A daily coffee or two can help protect against heart disease and boost metabolism. But be aware that the high levels of sugar/dairy in takeaway drinks like lattes and frappés might counteract coffee's benefits, so keep things simple by either enjoying it black or keeping any added dairy or sugar to a minimum. Regular consumption of tea (including black, green or herbal) has also been linked to a longer life, reduced risk of heart disease and reduced stress. Certain types of herbal teas can also help to soothe minor health complaints, encourage restful sleep and boost your immune system.

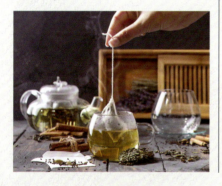

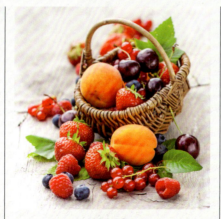

FRUITS

Fruits make a delicious, healthy choice for daily desserts and snacks. As with vegetables, you should aim to include several daily portions of fruit in your diet to enjoy a wide range of vitamins and minerals. 'Eat the rainbow' is a good rule of thumb to ensure variety, so pick different colours of fruit (and veg) when you shop. Choose fresh and seasonal fruits where possible, although frozen or tinned options are suitable alternatives. However, watch out for any tinned fruit that's steeped in syrup to avoid unnecessary added sugar. Whole fruits are better than juices, because you will get all the beneficial fibre.

NUTS & SEEDS

Packed full of healthy unsaturated fats, vitamins and minerals, nuts and seeds are nutritional powerhouses. Each type has different benefits – for example, just a small handful of walnuts contains your full daily recommended omega-3 fatty acids, while sesame seeds are rich in B vitamins, iron and magnesium. Nuts and seeds make a great snack on their own, but they are also wonderfully versatile: they work well in both sweet and savoury dishes; they can be toasted to deepen their flavour; blitzed into flours, nut butters and pastes (like tahini); and even soaked and blended to make homemade nut milks.

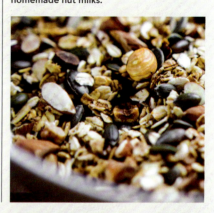

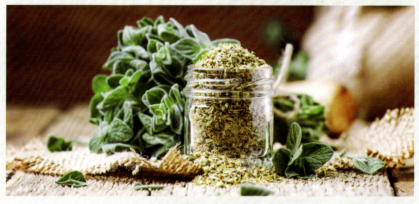

HERBS & SPICES

From the herbs of Provence to the fragrant spices of Morocco, Mediterranean meals will often feature one or more of these flavour-packed seasonings. Not only can herbs and spices make dishes extra tasty, but some of them have health-boosting properties too. For example, oregano is high in antioxidants and vitamin K, and may also help to reduce inflammation in the body, while cinnamon can help to regulate blood sugar levels and may also boost the 'good' bacteria in our guts. Even the kitchen staple of black pepper may help reduce cholesterol levels and improve the absorption of other nutrients in the body.

INTRODUCTION

WHAT TO HAVE IN MODERATION

THESE FOODS SHOULD SUPPLEMENT THE CORE COMPONENTS OF THE DIET OUTLINED ON PAGES 22-23. THEY CAN BE ENJOYED IN MODEST REGULAR SERVINGS, OR LARGER MONTHLY PORTIONS

FISH & SEAFOOD

Compared to a standard Western diet, fish and seafood are eaten more regularly on a Mediterranean diet. Aim for two or three portions weekly, with at least one being an oily fish like salmon or mackerel. Oily fishes are rich in omega-3 fatty acids, which are beneficial for heart and brain health.

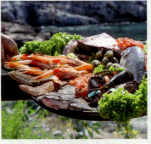

POULTRY

While fish is the main animal protein in a Mediterranean diet, poultry can also be eaten in moderate amounts – meat should supplement a meal rather than be the main event. Aim for one or two portions of poultry each week, and buy the highest-quality/welfare meat that your budget will allow.

DAIRY PRODUCTS

Dairy products like milk, yoghurt and cheese are still on the menu, but stick to small, daily portions or larger, weekly portions to avoid regularly over-indulging. Full-fat dairy is closer to the traditional eating habits the diet is based on, compared to modern low-fat options that may contain added sugar.

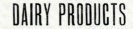

EGGS

Eggs are a wonderful source of high-quality protein and vitamins A, D, B2 and B12. Although the yolks contain cholesterol, studies have shown that this does not cause the same negative effects that eating saturated fat does, so enjoy the whole egg. An average of one egg per day is recommended.

RED MEAT

Beef, pork, lamb and other red meats should only be enjoyed occasionally. This could be small portions to flavour a dish or larger portions a couple of times a month. The regular consumption of red meat (particularly processed meat) has been found to increase the risk of cardiovascular disease.

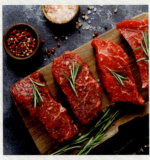

DESSERTS & SWEETS

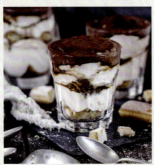

Fruit should be your go-to sweet snack or dessert, but you are still able to enjoy cakes and pastries. However, these should be enjoyed in moderation just a few times a month or saved for special occasions, rather than everyday indulgences.

RED WINE

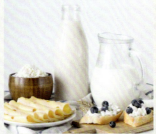
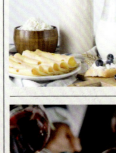

Red wine is rich in powerful antioxidants called polyphenols, which help to prevent or reverse cell damage in the body and can therefore help protect you against disease. Studies have found that drinking red wine in moderation – a small glass or two per day with meals – is linked to lower blood pressure, lower levels of inflammation, and even a lower risk of depression. If you don't drink wine, you can get similar benefits from dark-skinned grapes in the form of juice (look for brands with no added sugar) and by eating the fruits themselves, which provides the added bonus of fibre.

WHAT TO AVOID

TO GET THE BEST HEALTH BENEFITS FROM THE MEDITERRANEAN DIET, THESE FOODS SHOULD IDEALLY BE AVOIDED ALTOGETHER. IF YOU DO INDULGE, DON'T MAKE IT A HABIT

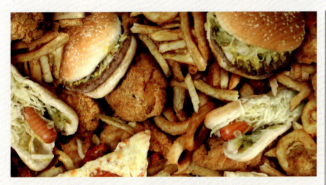

CONVENIENCE & 'JUNK' FOOD

A huge part of the Mediterranean diet and broader lifestyle is the idea that meals should be cooked from scratch and savoured. The concept of fast food, eating on-the-go, takeaways and microwave meals goes against the spirit of the Mediterranean approach. Junk foods in particular are often high in saturated fats and/or sugar, which should be avoided in this eating plan. However, the pace of modern life can make convenience foods inevitable at times; use your judgement and opt for the best option available to you – choose a supermarket vegetable pasta salad for lunch rather than a buttery bacon sandwich, for example.

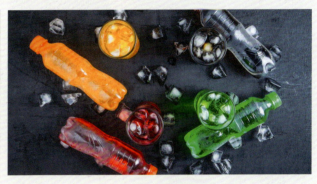

FIZZY DRINKS

High-sugar sodas play havoc with the body's blood sugar levels – some brands contain the equivalent of nine teaspoons of sugar in a single can. Regular consumption of fizzy drinks can lead to a variety of health problems, including increased risk of obesity, diabetes and tooth decay. 'Diet' versions may not contain any sugar, but studies suggest that the artificial sweeteners they use instead can harm the good bacteria in our guts, and may also negatively affect the body's metabolism. Energy drinks should be avoided for the same reasons, along with the potentially detrimental effects of their excessive caffeine content.

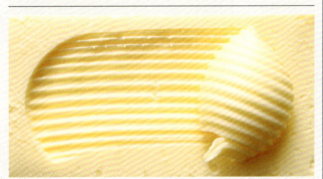

BUTTER

Butter is very high in saturated fat, which is linked to an increased risk of heart disease. Historically, butter was more commonly used in Northern Europe, whereas the Southern Europeans used olive oil. Butter would have been rarely used – if at all – in a traditional Mediterranean diet. This should be fairly easy to avoid, as olive oil will take its place in most of your cooking. You can also find olive oil spreads, but be sure to check the ingredients lists as some brands contain a mixture of other vegetable oils, or a blend of butter and olive oil.

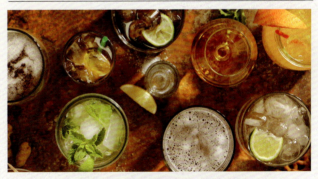

OTHER ALCOHOLIC DRINKS

While moderate consumption of red wine is allowed on a Mediterranean diet, other alcoholic drinks such as beers, ciders, spirits and cocktails are best avoided. Studies have shown that beers, spirits and white wine (which is made without the antioxidant-packed grape skins) do not appear to have the same health benefits as red wine. Drinks like ciders, spirits with mixers, liqueurs and cocktails are also typically high in sugar, and therefore pose a similar problem to fizzy drinks as mentioned above. If you are going to have a drink, always do so in moderation and with meals.

INTRODUCTION

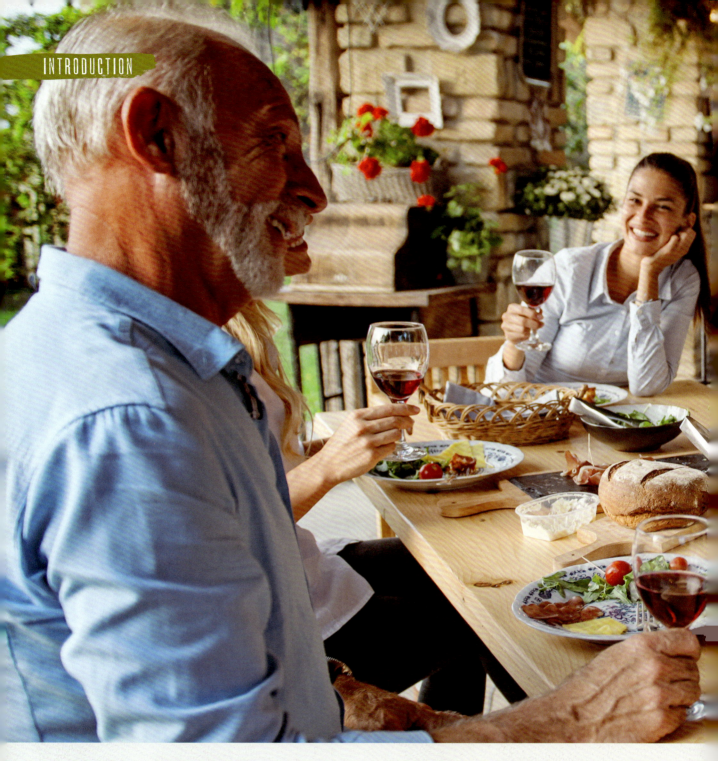

THE MEDITERRANEAN LIFESTYLE

BEYOND THE BENEFITS OF THE DIET ITSELF, EMBRACING OTHER TRADITIONAL
MEDITERRANEAN HABITS CAN HELP YOU LIVE A LONGER, HEALTHIER AND HAPPIER LIFE

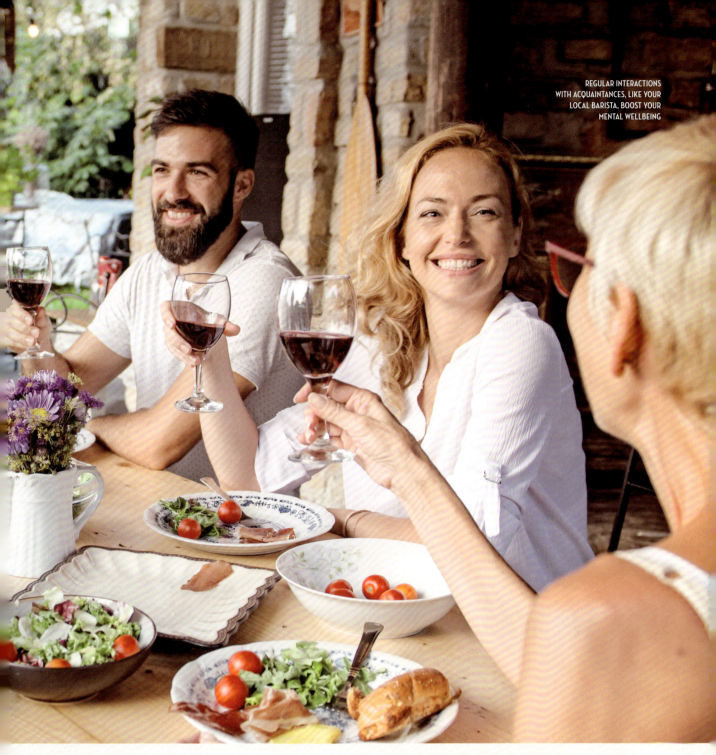

REGULAR INTERACTIONS WITH ACQUAINTANCES, LIKE YOUR LOCAL BARISTA, BOOST YOUR MENTAL WELLBEING

The Mediterranean diet has been scientifically proven to promote good health, but adopting a Mediterranean approach in other aspects of your life can also have a significant positive impact on your physical and mental wellbeing.

SOCIALISING & COMMUNITY SPIRIT

Regular socialising is a cornerstone of the Mediterranean lifestyle. Research has shown that having strong social bonds promotes good quality of life and mental health. For example, people who frequently socialise have a lower risk of hypertension and depression. Family life and friendship are at the heart of Mediterranean life, but it may surprise you to learn that even our relationships with casual acquaintances (known as 'weak ties') are beneficial too, as they foster a greater sense of belonging and community spirit. Studies have shown that older adults with a diverse network of weak ties and close ties (family and friends) enjoy a better quality of life and live longer than those with narrower social circles.

MAKE THE MOST OF MEALTIMES

It's not just what you eat, but *how*. Mediterranean mealtimes are a social

INTRODUCTION

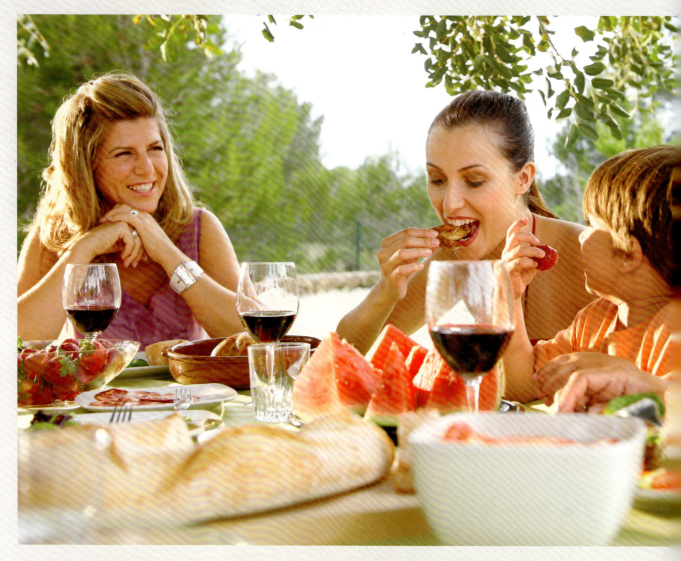

occasion and a welcome chance to spend time with family and friends. How many of us are guilty of having a hurried lunch 'al desko' or eating dinner in front of the television? Try to make time to really savour and enjoy your meals properly, whether that means taking your office lunch to the park with a book, eating together with colleagues, or sitting up at the dinner table together as a family. Allowing yourself time to appreciate both your food and company brings a range of benefits. Not only do we get the perks of socialising, but as conversation flows we naturally tend to eat more slowly when dining with others, which is better for your digestion. Spending quality time with others and taking breaks from the various stresses of the day is also hugely important for our mental health.

STAY ACTIVE

The benefits of regular exercise are well established, but keeping fit doesn't mean that you have to dedicate an hour every day to a strenuous high-intensity workout at the gym. Traditional Mediterranean communities naturally got their exercise as part of their daily routines, such as walking to town or through physical work like farming and fishing. Moderate, regular exercise is all that's needed to maintain a good level of fitness, as long as it gets your heart rate up. The 'best' exercise is anything that's easy to incorporate into your daily life and – most importantly – something you enjoy doing. That way you're more likely to stick at it. So whether it's swimming, a dance class, yoga or a brisk walk, aim for five to ten hours of physical activity each week.

> **MEDITERRANEAN MEALTIMES ARE A SOCIAL OCCASION AND A WELCOME CHANCE TO SPEND TIME WITH FAMILY AND FRIENDS**

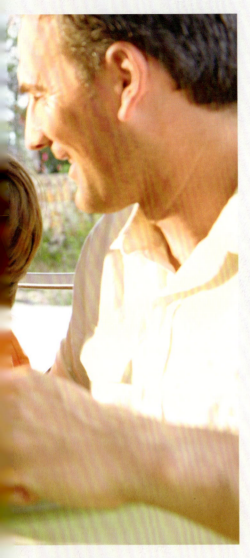

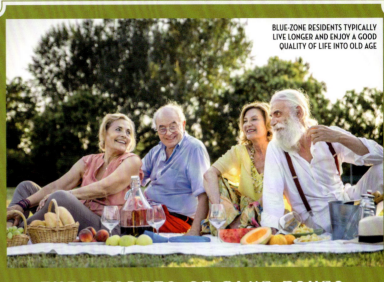

BLUE-ZONE RESIDENTS TYPICALLY LIVE LONGER AND ENJOY A GOOD QUALITY OF LIFE INTO OLD AGE

THE SECRETS OF BLUE ZONES

The Mediterranean contains two of the five regions known as 'Blue Zones': the Italian island of Sardinia and the Greek island of Ikaria. Blue Zones were identified during a *National Geographic* investigation into longevity, and also include Okinawa in Japan, Nicoya in Costa Rica and a religious community in Loma Linda, California. In these parts of the world, locals consistently live longer than the general population, with unusually high rates of people living well into their 90s and beyond – yet there are relatively low incidences of age-related diseases like dementia.

Researchers have since studied the lifestyles of Blue Zone populations in an attempt to understand this phenomenon. While diet is believed to be a major factor, other common characteristics include a strong focus on family and community, regular social contact and a moderately active lifestyle.

The most important thing the researchers learned, however, was that the healthy choices these people made were the easiest options available to them. For example, fresh produce was often more readily available than high-fat/sugar processed foods. The Blue Zones Project has used these findings as a model to help communities elsewhere enjoy similar benefits via local policy changes and education drives, making it easier for people to make healthy choices.

GET OUTDOORS

Not all of us are able to enjoy the balmy temperatures and sunshine of the Mediterranean, but getting outside and enjoying nature is still important no matter where you live. Modern life has led to us spending far more time indoors, but studies have shown that being in nature is beneficial to our mental health as it can help reduce stress, anxiety and depression. Regular exposure to sunlight is also an important source of vitamin D, which plays a vital role in keeping our bones, teeth and muscles healthy. Most people will get enough vitamin D in the summer months by being out in the sunshine for brief periods of time with forearms or lower legs uncovered (follow health advice and use sunscreen or cover up to avoid burning). Depending on where in the world you are, it may be more difficult to get enough vitamin D from sunlight alone in the winter months. Vitamin D is found in oily fish, eggs and red meat, but it may be difficult to get enough from food alone while following a Mediterranean diet, so consider speaking to your doctor about taking supplements to top up your levels.

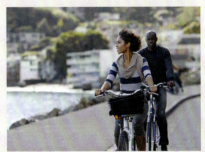

TAKING REGULAR EXERCISE AND ENJOYING NATURE ARE IMPORTANT ELEMENTS IN ANY HEALTHY LIFESTYLE

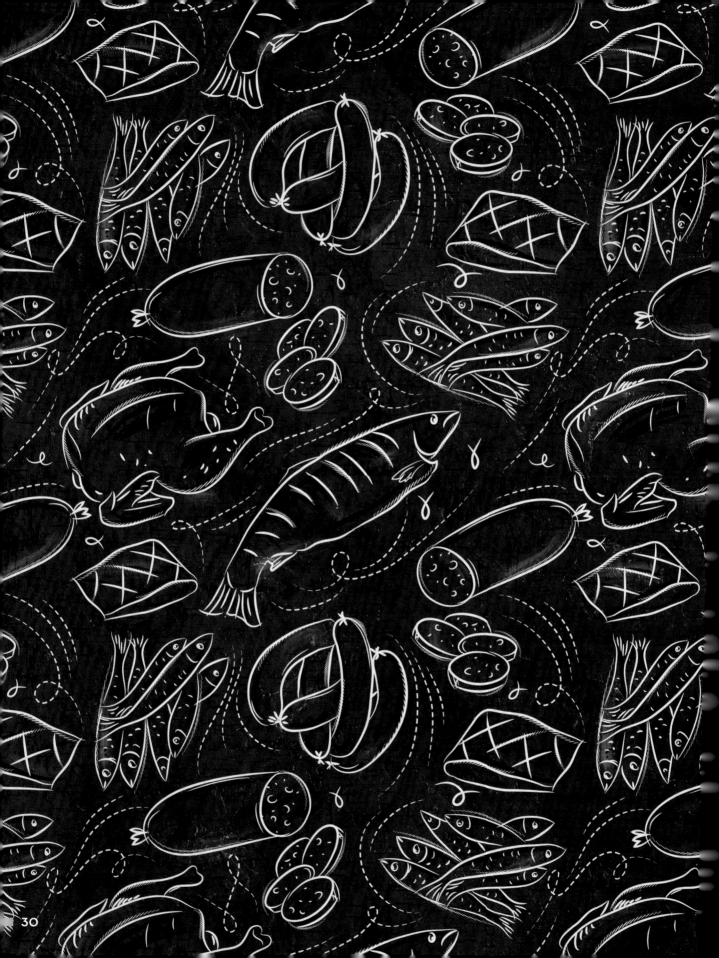

LIGHT BITES

Quilted olive and halloumi loaf	33
Mediterranean stuffed pepper	35
Watermelon, mint and feta salad	37
Ham and manchego croquettes	39
Sicilian caponata salad	41
Veggie frittata with Padrón peppers and greens	43
Tomato bread with anchovies	45
Gambas with aioli	47
Fig and goat's cheese puffs	49
Mediterranean layered sandwiches	51
Roasted Med veg and feta	53
Spanish chicken skewers and patatas bravas	55
Arty pepper focaccia	57
Mediterranean gratin	59
Watermelon 'pizza' with feta	61
Squid salad with garlic and chilli	63
Spanakopita	65
Hummus	67
Tabbouleh	69
Spanish omelette with saffron aioli	71
Burrata, bresaola and clementine salad	73
Baked feta Greek salad with figs	75
Roasted pepper and garlic bruschetta	77
Lamb arancini	79
Halloumi with a chilli kick	81
Baked stuffed tomatoes with harissa rice	83
Lamb pitta bites	85
Baba ganoush	87
Pissaladière	89
Polenta bread with antipasti	91

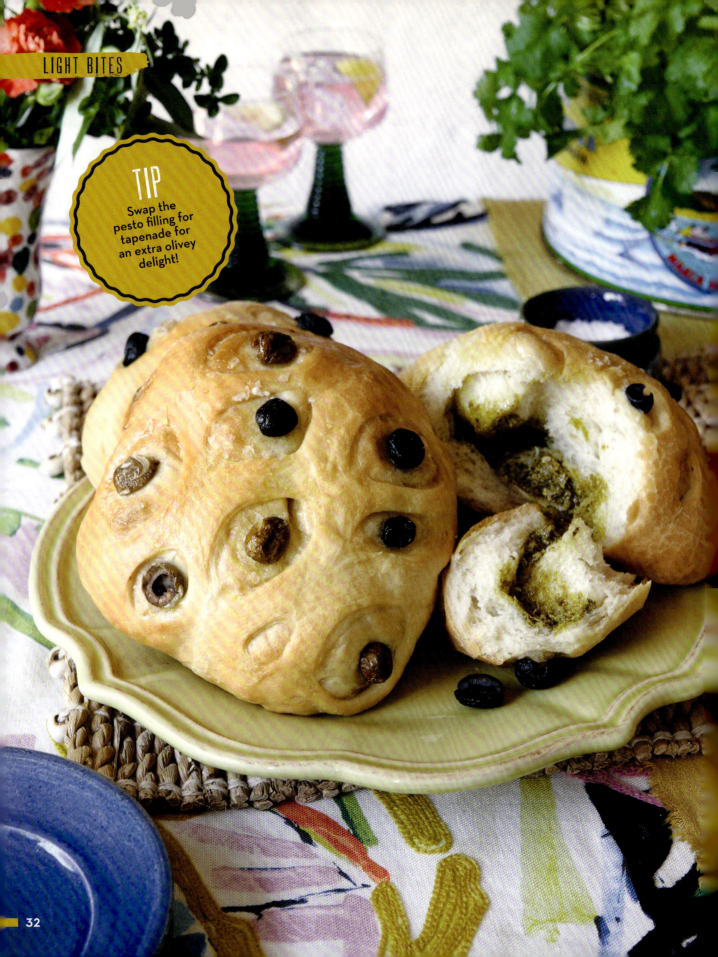

SERVINGS 4 | PREP TIME 30-40 MINS | REST TIME 1 HR 30 MINS | COOK TIME 20 MINS

QUILTED OLIVE AND HALLOUMI LOAF

THESE REGAL, PUFFY LOAVES ARE THE PERFECT ACCOMPANIMENT TO A MEDITERRANEAN SPREAD, AS THEY ARE MADE FOR SHARING AND TEARING

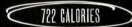

722 CALORIES

INGREDIENTS

- 500g | 17.6oz STRONG BREAD FLOUR
- 7g | 0.2oz DRIED YEAST OR 14g | 0.4oz FRESH YEAST
- 4tbsp OLIVE OIL, PLUS EXTRA FOR GREASING
- 2tsp SEA SALT
- 100g | 3.5oz HALLOUMI, CUT INTO 4 SLICES
- 4tsp PESTO
- 1 EGG, BEATEN
- 150g | 5.3oz PITTED OLIVES, ANY COLOUR

STEP 1 Tip the flour into a bowl and stir in the yeast. Add 300ml | 10floz lukewarm water and combine to form a dough. Add the olive oil and salt, and then knead the dough, either in a mixer with a dough hook, or on a lightly floured surface, for 8-10 mins until smooth and elastic.

STEP 2 Put the dough into an oiled bowl and smother the top with a little more oil. Cover with a clean damp tea towel and leave in a warm place to prove for 1 hr or until almost doubled in size.

STEP 3 Divide the dough into 6 pieces. Then divide 2 of the pieces in half again. Shape the 4 large pieces into flat discs, and place a slice of halloumi and 1tsp pesto into the centre of each disc. Fold the dough over, pinching the seams firmly together.

STEP 4 Place the 4 larger pieces of dough on a flour-dusted baking tray. Put a damp cloth on top and prove for a further 30 mins. Cover the smaller pieces in cling film and place in the fridge.

STEP 5 Preheat the oven to 220°C (200°C fan) | 425°F | gas 7. On a floured cutting board, roll the smaller dough pieces into 15cm | 6" rounds. Create a lattice pattern by making alternating incisions with a sharp knife.

STEP 6 Brush the halloumi-filled rolls with the egg. Stretch a smaller piece of dough over each to expose the holes and tuck the edges underneath. Press half an olive into each gap.

STEP 7 Cook the rolls for 20 mins. Serve them warm.

LIGHT BITES

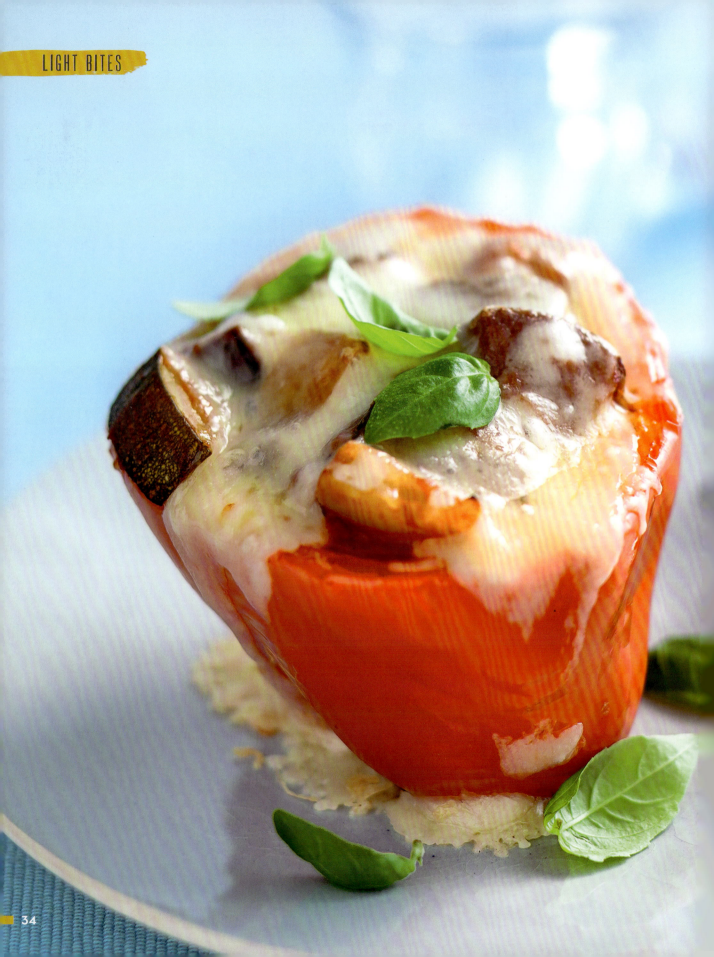

SERVINGS 1 | **PREP TIME 5 MINS** | **COOK TIME 25 MINS**

MEDITERRANEAN STUFFED PEPPER

USING LEFTOVER RATATOUILLE, THIS MAKES THE PERFECT LIGHT MEAL FOR WHEN YOU HAVEN'T GOT A LOT OF TIME TO PREP!

181 CALORIES

INGREDIENTS

- 1 SMALL RED BELL PEPPER
- 100G | 3.5OZ RATATOUILLE (SEE PAGE 105)
- 20G | 0.7OZ MATURE CHEESE (OPTIONAL)
- A FEW SMALL BASIL LEAVES

STEP 1 Cut the top off the pepper and scoop out the seeds. Place it in a shallow ovenproof dish, spoon the ratatouille into the pepper.

STEP 2 Preheat the oven to 200°C (180°C fan) | 400°F | gas 6. Bake the pepper for 20 mins or until the pepper is cooked.

STEP 3 If using, sprinkle the cheese over the stuffed pepper and return to the oven for 5 mins or until the cheese starts to melt and brown. Garnish with the basil leaves.

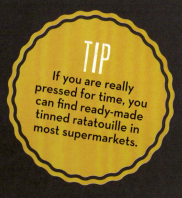

TIP
If you are really pressed for time, you can find ready-made tinned ratatouille in most supermarkets.

LIGHT BITES

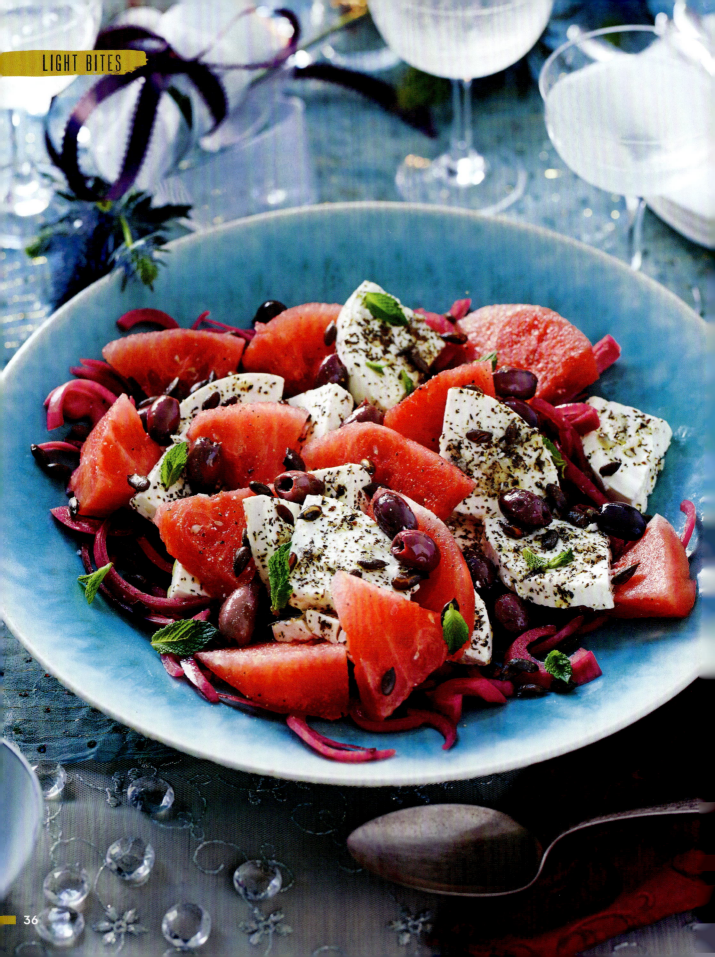

SERVINGS 8-12   PREP TIME 30 MINS   MARINATING TIME 4 HRS - OVERNIGHT

WATERMELON, MINT AND FETA SALAD

WE'VE USED TURKISH FETA IN THIS SALAD BUT THE GREEK VARIETY WILL WORK JUST AS WELL – IT'S JUST LESS CREAMY

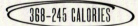

368-245 CALORIES

INGREDIENTS

- 2 RED ONIONS, FINELY SLICED
- 4 TBSP RED WINE VINEGAR
- 3 TBSP CASTER SUGAR
- 150ML | 5FLOZ EXTRA VIRGIN OLIVE OIL
- 2 GARLIC CLOVES, CRUSHED
- 1 TBSP DRIED MINT
- 450G | 16OZ FETA CHEESE, CUT INTO TRIANGLES (OPTIONAL, SEE TIP)
- 4 TBSP PUMPKIN SEEDS
- SEA SALT AND FRESHLY GROUND PEPPER
- 1 WATERMELON, CUT INTO TRIANGLES
- 100G | 3.5OZ PITTED BLACK OLIVES
- A FEW SPRIGS FRESH MINT, TO SERVE

STEP 1 Mix the onions with the vinegar and sugar. Stir well and set aside. Mix the olive oil with the garlic and dried mint. If using, carefully spread out the feta in a shallow dish, pour over the oil mixture and cover with cling film. Leave to marinate for at least 4 hrs or overnight.

STEP 2 Preheat the oven to 180°C (160°C fan) | 350°F | gas 4. Toss the pumpkin seeds with sea salt, black pepper and a little oil, and bake for 15 mins or until just starting to brown. Drain on kitchen paper.

STEP 3 When you're ready to serve, drain the onions and spread over a large, shallow dish. Top with feta (if using), interspersing the slices with watermelon. Spoon over the olive oil marinade then sprinkle over the pumpkin seeds and olives, and add a few sprigs of fresh mint.

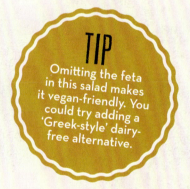

TIP Omitting the feta in this salad makes it vegan-friendly. You could try adding a 'Greek-style' dairy-free alternative.

LIGHT BITES

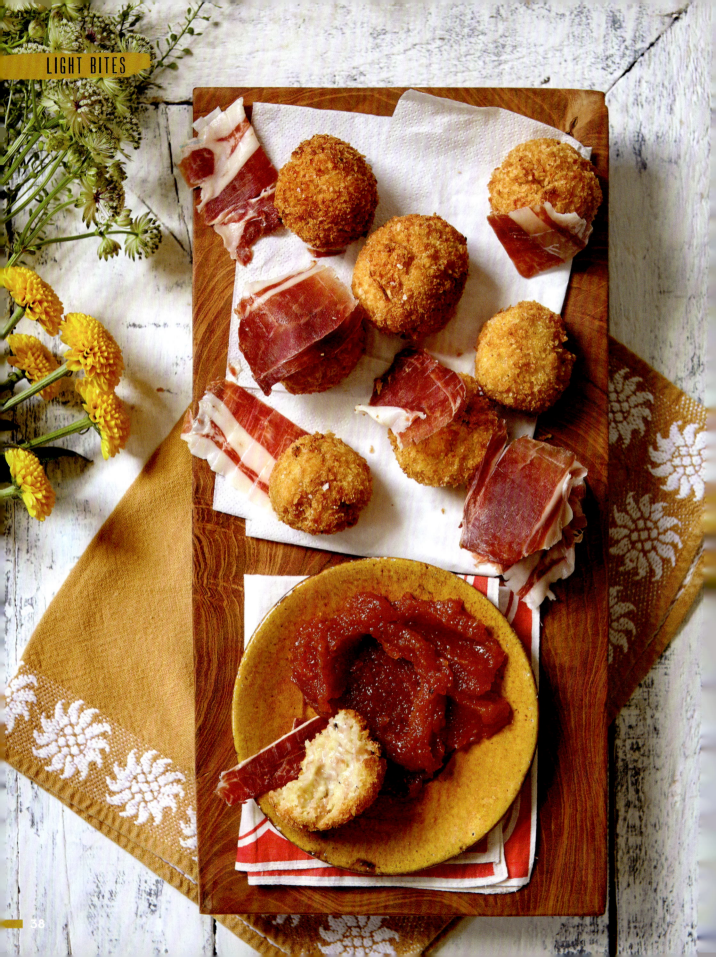

MAKES 20-24 | **PREP TIME 15-20 MINS** | **CHILL TIME 1 HR 45 MINS** | **COOK TIME 10-12 MINS**

HAM AND MANCHEGO CROQUETTES

THESE ARE UTTERLY MOREISH – PREPARE AHEAD AND POP IN THE OVEN TO REHEAT

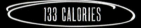

133 CALORIES

INGREDIENTS

4TBSP OLIVE OIL, PLUS PLENTY MORE FOR DEEP FRYING
1 SHALLOT
70G | 2.5OZ IBÉRICO HAM, DICED VERY SMALL, PLUS 70G | 2.5OZ EXTRA TO SERVE
100G | 3.5OZ PLAIN FLOUR
75ML | 2.5FLOZ VEGETABLE STOCK
325ML | 11FLOZ MILK
50G | 1.8OZ MANCHEGO CHEESE, GRATED
QUINCE PASTE, TO SERVE

FOR THE CRUMB:
75G | 2.6OZ PLAIN FLOUR
2 LARGE EGGS, BEATEN
100G | 3.5OZ BREADCRUMBS (WE HAVE USED PANKO CRUMBS)

STEP 1 Heat the oil in a pan, add the shallot, and sauté until soft but not coloured. Stir in the diced ham, fry for 1 min, then add the flour and fry over a medium heat until the mixture is golden.

STEP 2 Heat the stock and milk in a small pan until hot but not boiling. Then gradually add this liquid to the roux, stirring all the time. Continue to cook for 5 mins until it thickens. Add the cheese and season with black pepper. Pour the sauce onto a small baking tray then cover with cling film. Leave it to cool then put it in the fridge for 1 hr.

STEP 3 For the crumb, put the flour, eggs and crumbs into 3 bowls. Dust your hands with flour, take some of the cheese mixture and roll it to a walnut-sized ball. Dust with flour, then roll in the egg and then the breadcrumbs. Put on a tray and chill for 30-45 mins.

STEP 4 If you have a deep-fat fryer, heat the oil to 175°C | 350°F and fry the croquettes for 2 mins. If not, heat the oil in a frying pan until it starts to shimmer, then add 3-4 croquettes at a time and fry until golden. You don't want them to cook too quickly otherwise the centre won't be hot enough. Serve warm with the slices of ham and quince paste.

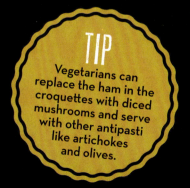

TIP
Vegetarians can replace the ham in the croquettes with diced mushrooms and serve with other antipasti like artichokes and olives.

LIGHT BITES

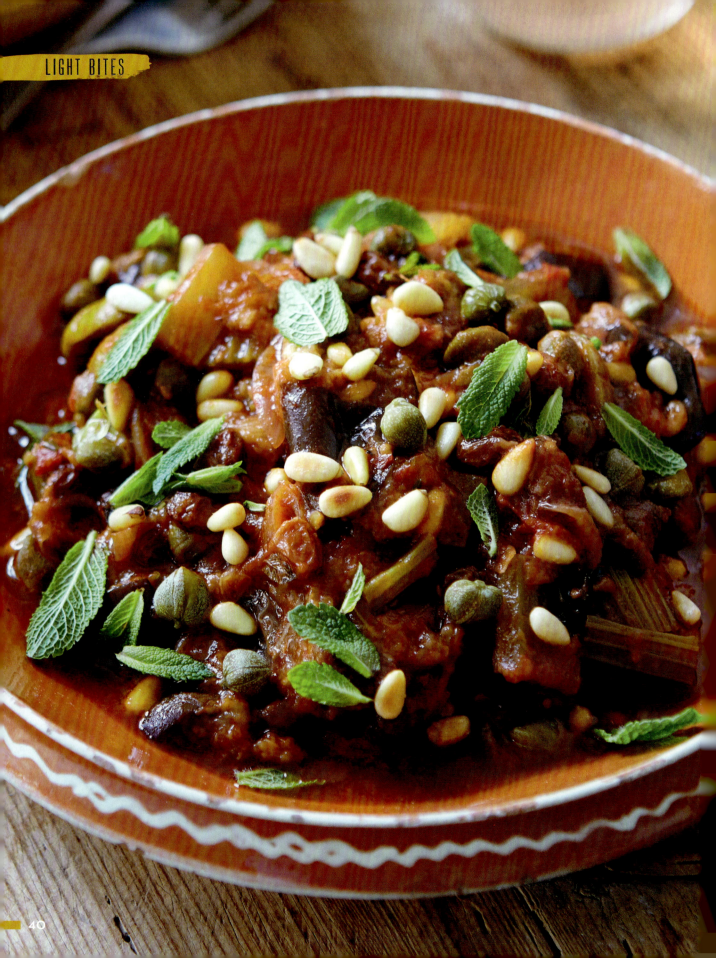

SERVINGS 8   PREP TIME 10-15 MINS   REST TIME 30 MINS   COOK TIME 50 MINS

SICILIAN CAPONATA SALAD

THIS SALAD, WITH ITS SWEET AND SOUR BALANCE OF FLAVOURS, IS A REAL ITALIAN CLASSIC

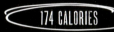

174 CALORIES

INGREDIENTS

- 2 LARGE AUBERGINES/EGGPLANTS, ABOUT 900G | 2LB, CUT INTO 2CM | 0.75" DICE
- SEA SALT AND FRESHLY GROUND PEPPER
- 3 TBSP OLIVE OIL, PLUS EXTRA FOR FRYING
- 1 LARGE RED ONION, SLICED
- 2 CELERY STICKS, CUT INTO 2CM | 0.75" DICE
- 2 RED BELL PEPPERS, SLICED
- 150G | 5.3OZ RIPE TOMATOES, DICED
- 40G | 1.4OZ CAPERS
- 40G | 1.4OZ PITTED GREEN OLIVES, QUARTERED
- 40G | 1.4OZ SULTANAS/GOLDEN RAISINS
- 1 TBSP SUGAR
- 50ML | 1.7FLOZ PASSATA/TOMATO PURÉE
- 100ML | 3.4FLOZ RED WINE VINEGAR
- 40G | 1.4OZ PINE NUTS, TOASTED, TO SERVE
- A SMALL BUNCH MINT OR BASIL, LEAVES ONLY, TO SERVE

STEP 1 Lightly salt the diced aubergine and leave for 30 mins in a colander over a sink, then pat dry. Heat a wide, deep pan one-third full of olive oil until it reaches 190°C | 375°F, or a cube of bread dropped in turns golden immediately. Fry the aubergine cubes in batches until golden. Allow the oil to reach that temperature again between each batch. Drain the aubergine on kitchen paper.

STEP 2 Heat the 3tbsp olive oil in a large, wide pan over a medium-low heat; cook the onion, celery and peppers with a pinch of salt until soft and beginning to colour. Cook for another min, then add the diced tomatoes and cook for another few mins.

STEP 3 Stir in the capers, olives, sultanas, sugar, passata and vinegar, bring to the boil, then add the fried aubergine. Season to taste, turn the heat right down and simmer gently for 30 mins. Remove from the heat and allow to cool. It tastes better made the day before serving and will keep for 5 days in the fridge, but allow it to come to room temperature before serving with the pine nuts and mint scattered over it.

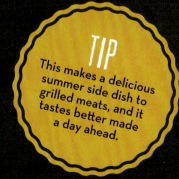

TIP
This makes a delicious summer side dish to grilled meats, and it tastes better made a day ahead.

LIGHT BITES

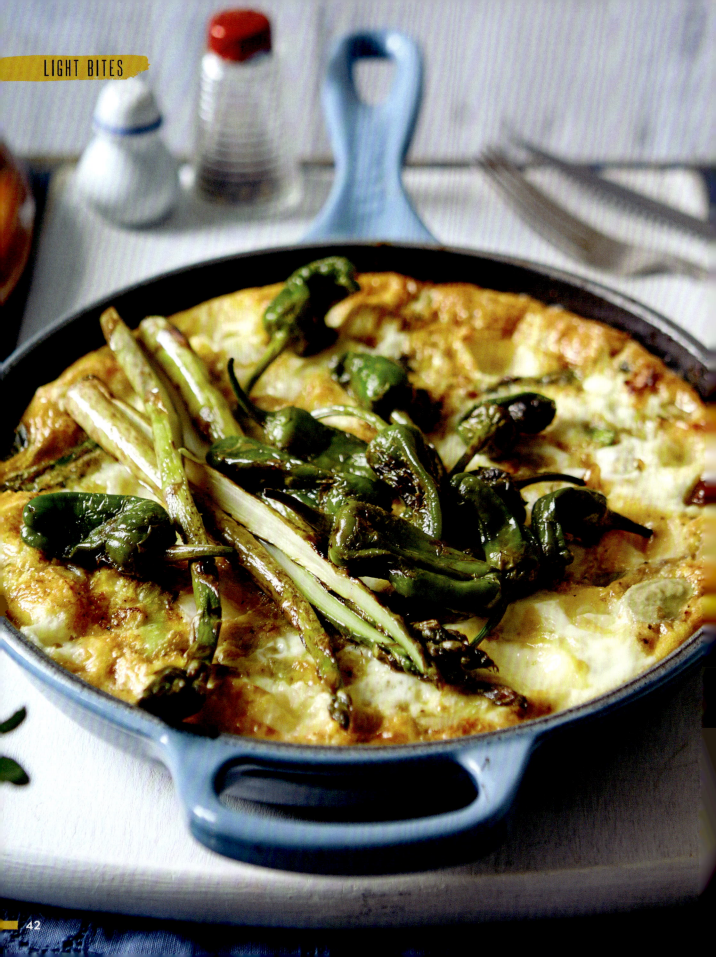

SERVINGS 10 | PREP TIME 5-10 MINS | COOK TIME 35 MINS

VEGGIE FRITTATA WITH PADRÓN PEPPERS AND GREENS

HAVE FUN GAMBLING WITH YOUR PADRÓN PEPPERS – ONE IN EVERY 20 IS SAID TO BE FIERY HOT!

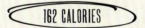

162 CALORIES

INGREDIENTS

1 TBSP OLIVE OIL
1 LEEK, SLICED INTO COINS
2 GARLIC CLOVES, CRUSHED
150G | 5.3OZ BROAD BEANS/FAVA BEANS
125G | 4.4OZ ASPARAGUS, CHOPPED INTO 5CM | 2" PIECES (RESERVE A FEW WHOLE)
A SMALL BUNCH EACH OF MINT AND BASIL, LEAVES ONLY, PLUS A FEW TO GARNISH
8 EGGS, BEATEN
150G | 5.3OZ MANCHEGO CHEESE, CUBED
130G | 4.5OZ PADRÓN PEPPERS
SEA SALT AND FRESHLY GROUND PEPPER

STEP 1 Preheat the oven to 190°C (170°C fan) | 375°F | gas 5. Heat the oil in an ovenproof frying pan and gently cook the leek and garlic for 5 mins until soft. Meanwhile, blanch the broad beans in boiling water for 2 mins.

STEP 2 Add the beans, asparagus, mint and basil to the frying pan and fry for a further 5 mins. Pour over the eggs and add the cheese. Cook over a low heat for 5 mins, until the eggs are half set. Transfer to the oven and cook for 10-15 mins.

STEP 3 While the frittata is cooking, heat a griddle pan to high and char the whole asparagus and Padrón peppers for a few mins. Sprinkle generously with salt and pepper. Serve the frittata with the reserved mint and basil leaves, the Padrón peppers and whole asparagus, plus a mixed leaf salad, if liked.

TIP
This dish can also be enjoyed at room temperature, so it makes a nutritious addition to a packed lunch.

LIGHT BITES

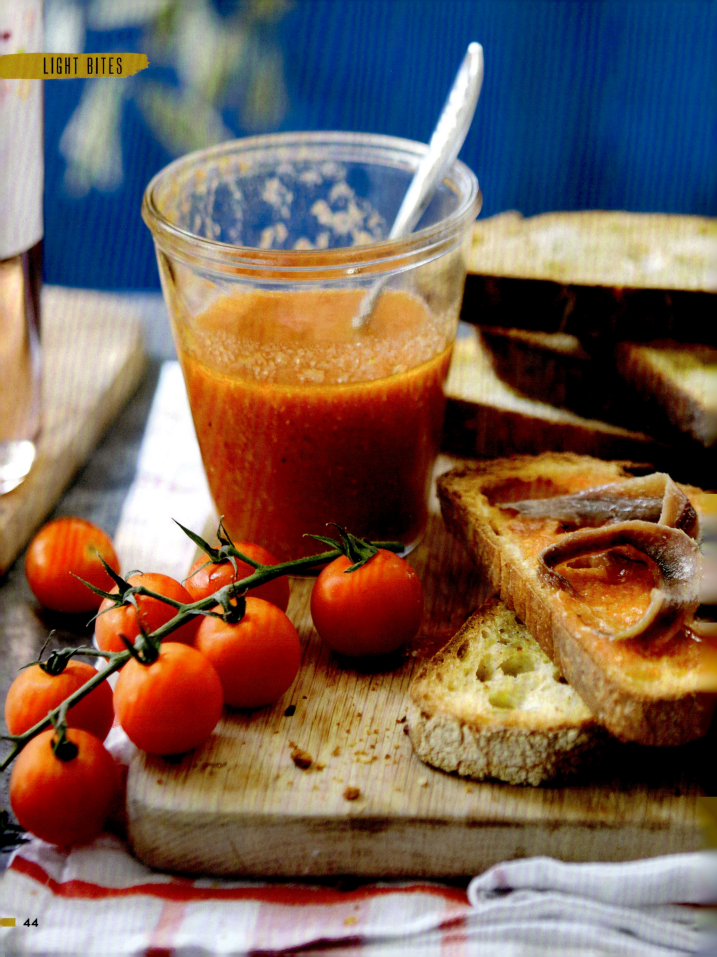

MAKES 400ML | 13.5FLOZ **COOK TIME 20-25 MINS**

TOMATO BREAD WITH ANCHOVIES

THIS QUICK AND EASY SAUCE IS A DELICIOUS SAUCE IN ITSELF, BUT HERE WE ARE USING IT AS A TASTY SPREAD

493 CALORIES

TIP
This recipe can also be made in bulk and frozen in portions. It can serve as a base for other tomato sauces, and goes well with pasta.

INGREDIENTS

100ML | 3.4FLOZ OLIVE OIL
5 GARLIC CLOVES
500G | 17.6OZ RIPE TOMATOES
SEA SALT AND FRESHLY GROUND PEPPER

TO SERVE, PER PERSON:
2 SLICES TOASTED SOURDOUGH BREAD
4 ANCHOVIES, FROM TINNED, DRAINED

STEP 1 Gently warm the oil in a large sauté pan. Add the garlic and allow this to infuse for 10 mins.

STEP 2 Add the tomatoes and leave them to cook gently until mushy. Put the whole mixture through a vegetable mill, potato ricer or colander to remove the skins. Season the sauce well with sea salt and black pepper.

STEP 3 To serve, spread 2tbsp sauce onto each slice of toasted bread and top with the anchovies. To store in the fridge, pour it into a sterilised jam jar and keep it well sealed.

This recipe is a take on pan con tomate, a simple Spanish tapas that can also be enjoyed as a savoury breakfast.

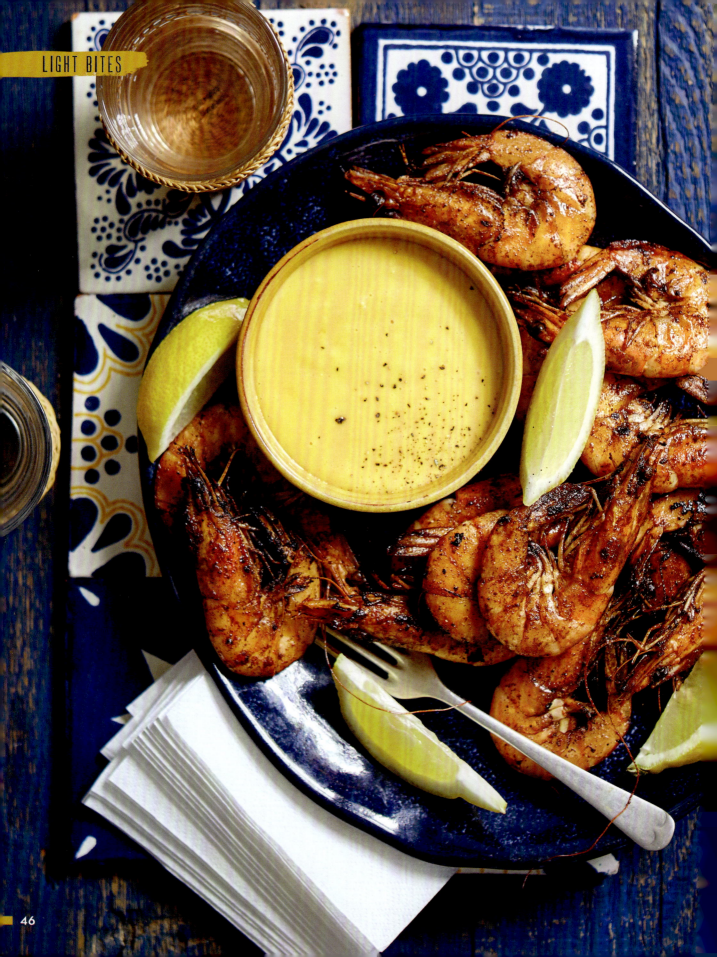
LIGHT BITES

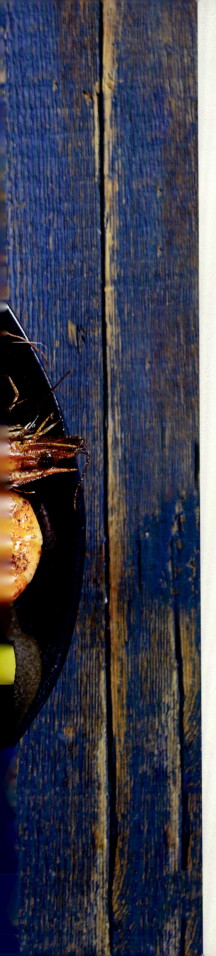

SERVINGS 6   PREP TIME 5–10 MINS   COOK TIME 5 MINS

GAMBAS WITH AIOLI

COOKING THE PRAWNS WITH THEIR SHELLS AND HEADS ON BOOSTS THE FLAVOUR OF THIS TAPAS CLASSIC

246 CALORIES

INGREDIENTS

- 18 PRAWNS, WITH HEAD AND SHELL ON
- 2 TSP SMOKED PAPRIKA
- 50ML | 1.7FLOZ OLIVE OIL
- 2 TBSP SHERRY VINEGAR
- 2 TBSP FLAT-LEAF/ITALIAN PARSLEY, CHOPPED, TO SERVE (OPTIONAL)
- LEMON WEDGES, TO SERVE

FOR THE AIOLI:
- 2 LARGE GARLIC CLOVES, CRUSHED
- ½ LEMON, JUICE ONLY
- 1 EGG YOLK, LIGHTLY WHISKED
- 125ML | 4.2FLOZ EXTRA VIRGIN OLIVE OIL

STEP 1 Toss the prawns with the paprika and set aside to marinate. For the aioli, place the garlic, lemon juice and egg yolk in a bowl. Slowly add the oil using an electric whisk until the mixture becomes thick and creamy. Check the seasoning and add more lemon juice or garlic if necessary, then set aside.

STEP 2 Heat the oil in a pan until hot and cook the prawns for 2–3 mins on each side, until almost cooked. Add the vinegar for the last 30 secs and cook it off.

STEP 3 Remove the prawns from the heat, top with parsley (if using) and serve with the lemon wedges and aioli.

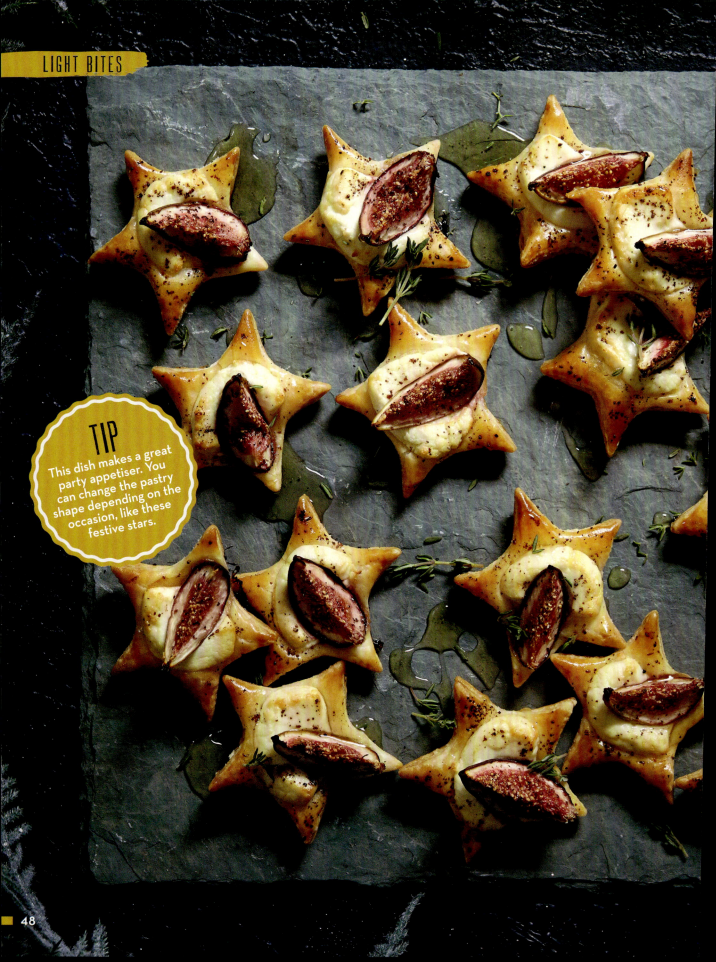

LIGHT BITES

TIP
This dish makes a great party appetiser. You can change the pastry shape depending on the occasion, like these festive stars.

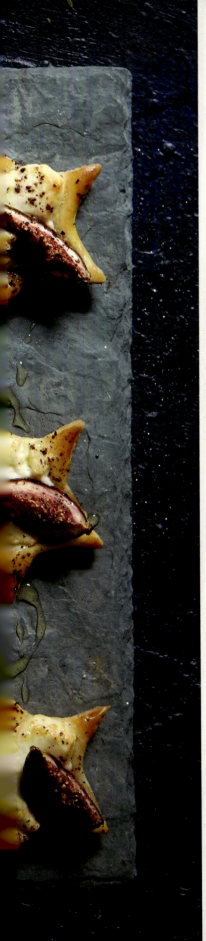

MAKES 20 PUFFS | PREP TIME 10 MINS | COOK TIME 30 MINS

FIG AND GOAT'S CHEESE PUFFS

A DELICIOUS COMBINATION OF CHEESE WITH THE SWEET TOUCH OF FIG AND HONEY MAKES THESE A MARVELLOUS MEDITERRANEAN MOUTHFUL

87 CALORIES

INGREDIENTS

320G | 11.3OZ READY-ROLLED PUFF PASTRY
1 EGG, BEATEN, FOR AN EGG WASH
1 LOG GOAT'S CHEESE, CUT INTO 18-20 HALF-MOON SHAPES
4 FIGS, EACH ONE CUT INTO 5 WEDGES
½ TSP SUMAC
A GENEROUS DRIZZLE OF HONEY
A FEW SPRIGS FRESH THYME, TO GARNISH

STEP 1 Preheat the oven to 180°C (160°C fan) | 350°F | gas 4. Use a cookie cutter in the design of your choice to cut out 10-12 shapes from the sheet of puff pastry and place them on a baking tray, leaving space between each one. Alternatively, you can use a knife to slice the pastry into 10-12 squares, about 8-10cm | 3-4" across.

STEP 2 Brush each piece of pastry with egg wash. Top with a piece of goat's cheese and a fig wedge. Sprinkle over the sumac and bake for 30 mins until the pastry is golden brown and cooked through.

STEP 3 Remove from the oven, drizzle with honey and garnish with thyme. Allow the puffs to cool slightly before serving.

LIGHT BITES

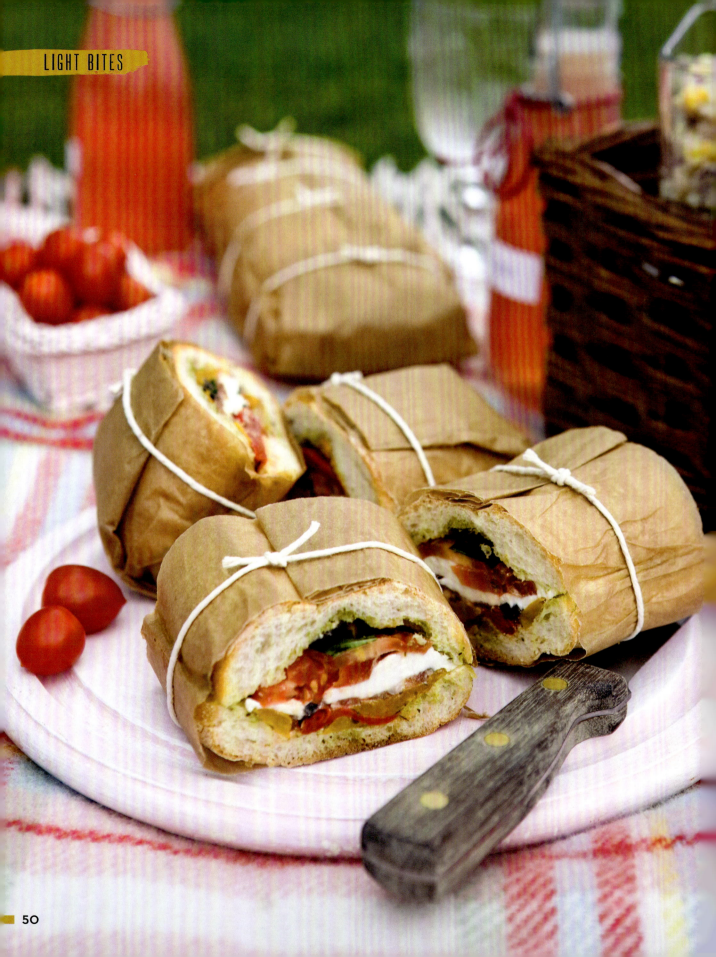

SERVINGS 8   PREP TIME 10 MINS

MEDITERRANEAN LAYERED SANDWICHES

PACKED WITH TASTY VEG AND OOZY MOZZARELLA, THESE CIABATTAS ARE GUARANTEED TO IMPRESS

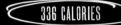
336 CALORIES

INGREDIENTS

- 2 CIABATTA LOAVES
- 1-2TBSP (LEVEL) BASIL PESTO
- 4TBSP EXTRA VIRGIN OLIVE OIL
- 2X 200G | 7OZ JARS ROASTED RED BELL PEPPERS, DRAINED
- 4 PLUM TOMATOES, SLICED
- 4-6TBSP PITTED BLACK OLIVES, SLICED
- FRESH BASIL LEAVES, TORN
- 2X 125G | 4.4OZ PACKETS MOZZARELLA, DRAINED AND SLICED

IF MAKING TO GO, YOU WILL NEED:
BAKING PAPER; STRING

STEP 1 Cut the ciabatta loaves in half lengthways. Mix the pesto and olive oil together, then brush this over the cut surfaces of the bread.

STEP 2 Use half of the rest of the ingredients for each loaf. Working on 1 loaf at a time, spread half the peppers over the bottom of the loaf, then arrange half the sliced plum tomatoes on top. Season, and add the olives and basil.

STEP 3 Top with the mozzarella slices then layer up the remaining ingredients in reverse order (ie torn basil, olives, tomato slices and then the peppers).

STEP 4 Place the top on the loaf, then wrap it in baking paper and tie tightly with string to hold it together. Fill the other loaf and wrap it in the same way.

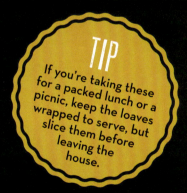

TIP
If you're taking these for a packed lunch or a picnic, keep the loaves wrapped to serve, but slice them before leaving the house.

LIGHT BITES

SERVINGS 1   PREP TIME 10 MINS   COOK TIME 15-20 MINS

ROASTED MED VEG AND FETA

THIS VEGGIE-FRIENDLY POT IS JUST THE THING FOR A SIMPLE AND SATISFYING PACKED LUNCH

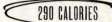

290 CALORIES

INGREDIENTS

- **200G | 7OZ** AUBERGINE/EGGPLANT, CUT INTO SMALL CHUNKS
- **200G | 7OZ** COURGETTE/ZUCCHINI, CUT INTO SMALL CHUNKS
- **1** SMALL RED ONION, CHOPPED
- A FEW LEAVES FRESH OREGANO OR THYME
- **2** GARLIC CLOVES, CRUSHED
- **1-2TSP** RAS EL HANOUT (TO TASTE)
- SEA SALT AND FRESHLY GROUND PEPPER
- EXTRA VIRGIN OLIVE OIL, TO DRIZZLE
- **1** LEMON, ZEST AND JUICE
- **2** HANDFULS BABY SPINACH
- A FEW LEAVES FRESH PARSLEY
- **50G | 1.8OZ** FETA CHEESE, CRUMBLED (OR **2TSP** MIXED SEEDS)

STEP 1 Preheat the oven to 200°C (180°C fan) | 400°F | gas 6. Toss together the aubergine, courgette, onion, oregano or thyme, garlic and ras el hanout, and season with salt and freshly ground black pepper. Spread out onto a lined baking tray and drizzle with the olive oil. Roast for 15-20 mins, or until golden brown. Scatter over the lemon zest and add a squeeze of juice. Leave to cool.

STEP 2 Put the cooked vegetables into the base of a Kilner or large screw-top jar. Place the spinach leaves on top with the parsley leaves and crumbled feta or seeds. Cover and chill until ready to eat.

TIP
The salty feta helps season the veggies, but you could swap it for a few Parmesan shavings.

LIGHT BITES

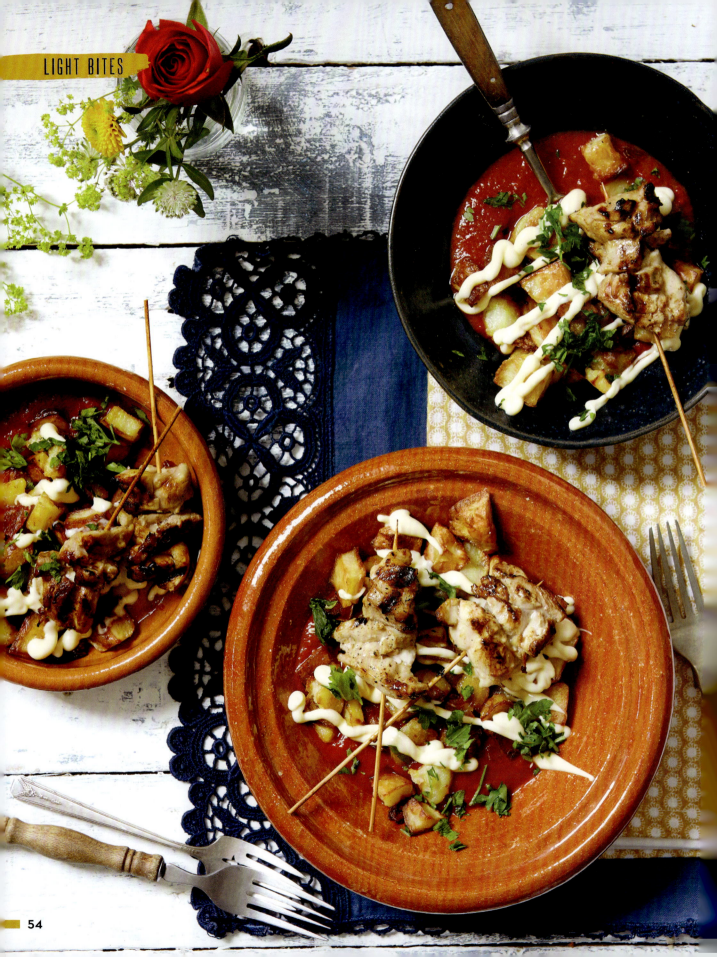

SERVINGS 8 | **PREP TIME 20 MINS** | **MARINATING TIME 30 MINS - OVERNIGHT** | **COOK TIME 1 HR 15 MINS**

SPANISH CHICKEN SKEWERS WITH PATATAS BRAVAS

THESE SIMPLE AND DELICIOUS SKEWERS ARE IDEAL FOR SHARING

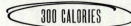

300 CALORIES

INGREDIENTS

FOR THE CHICKEN:
- 8 SKINLESS, BONELESS CHICKEN THIGHS, CUT INTO 3CM | 1" PIECES
- 2TBSP OLIVE OIL
- 4 GARLIC CLOVES, CRUSHED
- 100ML | 3.4FLOZ DRY SHERRY
- 2TBSP HONEY

FOR THE PATATAS BRAVAS:
- 5TBSP OLIVE OIL
- 1KG | 2.2LB WAXY POTATOES, PEELED AND CUT INTO 2CM | 0.75" CHUNKS
- 2 GARLIC CLOVES, CRUSHED
- ½ RED CHILLI, FINELY CHOPPED
- 250G | 8.8OZ PASSATA/ TOMATO PURÉE
- ½ TBSP TOMATO PURÉE/PASTE
- 1TBSP SHERRY VINEGAR
- 1TSP PAPRIKA (SMOKED OR SWEET)
- ½ TSP CASTER SUGAR
- MAYONNAISE, TO SERVE (OPTIONAL)

YOU WILL NEED:
- 8 LONG WOODEN SKEWERS, SOAKED IN WATER FOR 1 HR

STEP 1 Toss the chicken pieces with the oil, garlic, sherry and honey. Marinate for 30 mins or overnight in the fridge.

STEP 2 Preheat the oven to 200°C (180°C fan) | 400°F | gas 6. For the patatas bravas, pour 3tbsp oil into a roasting tray and heat for 10 mins, then toss the potatoes in it and season. Roast for 50 mins, turning halfway through, until golden and really crispy.

STEP 3 Heat the remaining oil in a pan and cook the garlic and chilli for 2 mins.

STEP 4 Add the passata, tomato purée, vinegar, paprika and sugar with plenty of seasoning and cook for 10 mins.

STEP 5 Meanwhile, thread the chicken onto the skewers and cook on a hot griddle pan or on the barbecue for 5-6 mins each side, until the chicken is cooked through and the edges are charred. You may need to finish the skewers off in the oven if some of the chicken is thicker.

STEP 6 To serve, spread the spicy tomato sauce over the base of a serving platter or individual plates, spread over the potatoes, drizzle with mayonnaise and top with chicken skewers.

LIGHT BITES

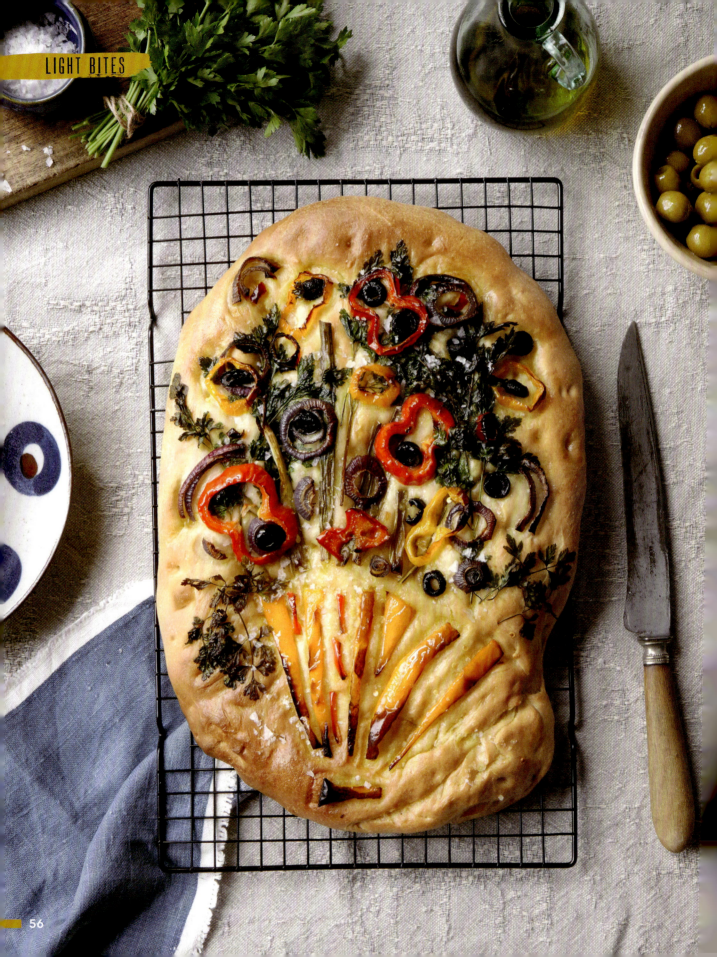

SERVINGS 10 **PREP TIME** 30 MINS **REST TIME** 1 HR 20-50 MINS **COOK TIME** 35 MINS

ARTY PEPPER FOCACCIA

LET THE DOUGH BE YOUR CANVAS AND TURN YOUR LOAF INTO SOMETHING SPECIAL WITH THIS CREATIVE BAKE

231 CALORIES

INGREDIENTS

- 500G | 17.6OZ STRONG BREAD FLOUR
- 7G | 0.2OZ SACHET FAST-ACTION DRIED YEAST, OR 14G | 0.4OZ FRESH YEAST
- 3TBSP OLIVE OIL, PLUS EXTRA FOR GREASING AND TO SERVE
- 2TSP SEA SALT, PLUS EXTRA TO SERVE

FOR THE DECORATION:
A SELECTION OF VEG AND HERBS THAT CAN BE EATEN RAW, SUCH AS:
- RED ONION
- PARSLEY
- BELL PEPPERS
- SPRING ONIONS/SCALLIONS
- OLIVES
- CHILLIES

YOU WILL NEED:
LARGE BAKING TRAY, LINED WITH BAKING PAPER

STEP 1 Tip the strong bread flour into a large bowl and stir in the yeast. Add 300ml | 10floz lukewarm water, the olive oil and sea salt, then mix to form a dough. Knead the dough, either in a mixer with a dough hook, or on a lightly floured surface, for 8-10 mins until smooth and elastic.

STEP 2 Put the dough into an oiled bowl and cover the top with a little more oil. Cover the bowl with cling film and leave in a warm place to prove for 60-90 mins until it has doubled in size.

STEP 3 Roll or stretch the dough out to a 35x25cm | 14x10" rectangle on a floured countertop. Place it on to the baking tray and make deep dimples with your fingers over the dough.

STEP 4 Artfully arrange the vegetables and herbs close together, to create an attractive pattern. Press them into the dough a little and brush over olive oil. Leave in a warm place for 20 mins. Meanwhile, preheat the oven to 200°C (180°C fan) | 400°F | gas 6.

STEP 5 Bake the bread for 15 mins, then brush or drizzle over a little more olive oil. Return to the oven for 20 mins and bake until golden.

STEP 6 Drizzle the loaf with a little more olive oil, plus a scattering of sea salt. It's best served warm.

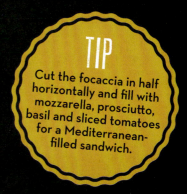

TIP
Cut the focaccia in half horizontally and fill with mozzarella, prosciutto, basil and sliced tomatoes for a Mediterranean-filled sandwich.

LIGHT BITES

SERVINGS 4 · PREP TIME 20 MINS · COOK TIME 30 MINS

MEDITERRANEAN GRATIN

THIS IS A PERFECT SUMMERY, VEGETABLE BAKE – DELICIOUS WITH CRUSTY BREAD AND A GLASS OF RED WINE

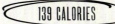

139 CALORIES

INGREDIENTS

- 1 RED BELL PEPPER
- 6 TOMATOES
- 2TBSP OLIVE OIL
- 1 RED ONION, FINELY SLICED
- 2 GARLIC CLOVES, CRUSHED
- 1TBSP MINT, CHOPPED
- 1TBSP BASIL, CHOPPED
- 1TBSP PARSLEY, CHOPPED
- 1-2 MEDIUM COURGETTES/ZUCCHINIS
- 50G | 1.8OZ CHEDDAR CHEESE, GRATED (OPTIONAL)

STEP 1 Cut the red pepper in half and discard the core. Dice the pepper and 2 tomatoes. Heat 1tbsp oil in a pan and fry the sliced onion, crushed garlic and diced pepper until tender. Add the chopped tomato and most of the herbs, then cook for 5 mins until softened.

STEP 2 Spoon half this mixture into a shallow gratin/baking dish. Preheat the oven to 180°C (160°C fan) | 350°F | gas 4.

STEP 3 Slice the courgettes and the remaining tomatoes and toss into the gratin/baking dish. Sprinkle over seasoning and add the remaining pepper mixture, then drizzle with the remaining oil.

STEP 4 Bake for 20 mins until the vegetables are almost tender, then sprinkle with the cheese (if using) and the rest of the herbs. Cook for a further 5 mins until the cheese has melted.

LIGHT BITES

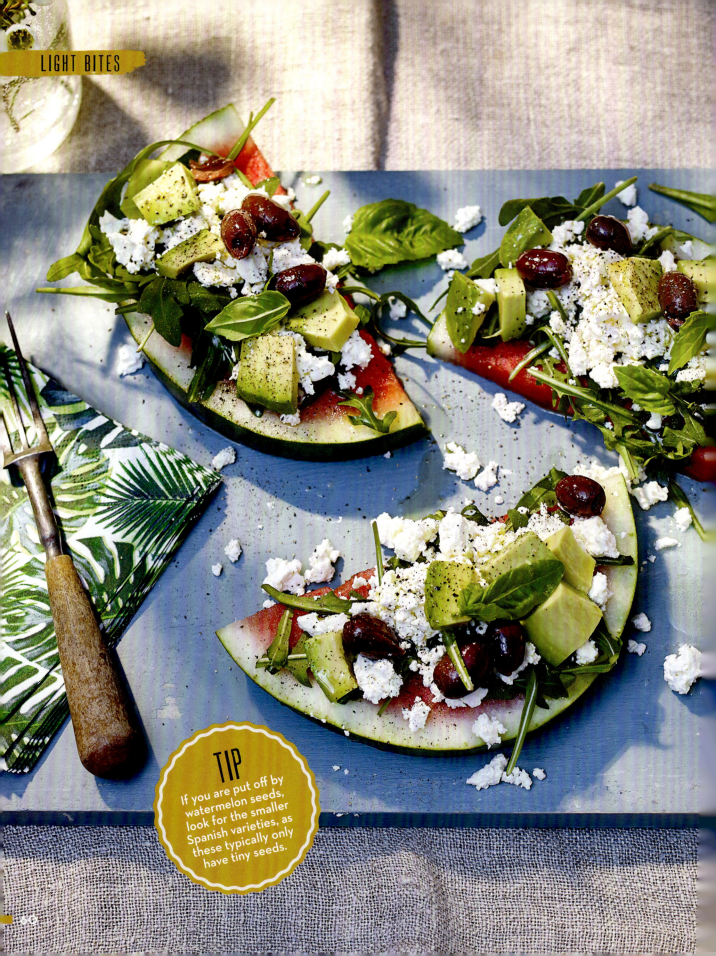

TIP
If you are put off by watermelon seeds, look for the smaller Spanish varieties, as these typically only have tiny seeds.

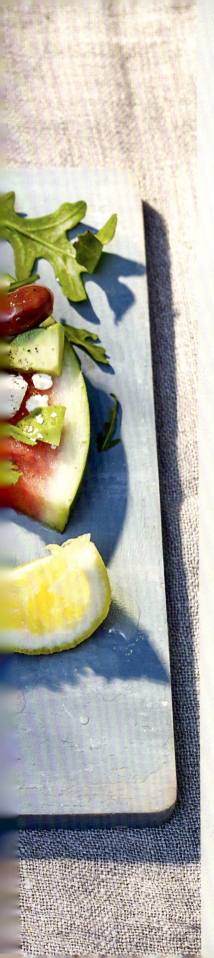

SERVINGS 4   PREP TIME 5-10 MINS

WATERMELON 'PIZZA' WITH FETA

THIS IS A FUN WAY TO SERVE A SALAD OR STARTER

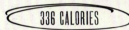

336 CALORIES

INGREDIENTS

2 SLICES WATERMELON (SEE TIP), ABOUT **2CM | 0.75"** THICK
2 HANDFULS SALAD LEAVES OF YOUR CHOICE, SUCH AS ROCKET/ARUGULA
100G | 3.5OZ FETA, CRUMBLED (OR GOAT'S CHEESE, OPTIONAL)
1 AVOCADO, PEELED, STONED AND DICED INTO SMALL CHUNKS
80G | 2.8OZ PITTED BLACK OLIVES
2TBSP EXTRA VIRGIN OLIVE OIL
FRESHLY GROUND BLACK PEPPER, TO TASTE
FRESH BASIL LEAVES, TO GARNISH
LEMON WEDGES, TO SERVE (OPTIONAL)

STEP 1 Halve each piece of watermelon to create 4 half-moons as your 'pizza' slices.

STEP 2 Top each slice with a quarter each of: the salad leaves, feta, avocado and olives. Drizzle the slices with olive oil, season generously with black pepper, and garnish with the basil leaves.

STEP 3 Serve immediately, with lemon wedges to squeeze over if using. This recipe can easily be doubled or tripled to serve larger groups. Experiment by mixing and matching other toppings to discover your favourite combination.

You can put whatever you like on top, but the watermelon and feta are the basic combination, with the sweetness of the fruit and the saltiness of the cheese.

LIGHT BITES

TIP
Don't be afraid of squid. Just cook it quickly on a super-hot barbecue or griddle pan and it won't be tough.

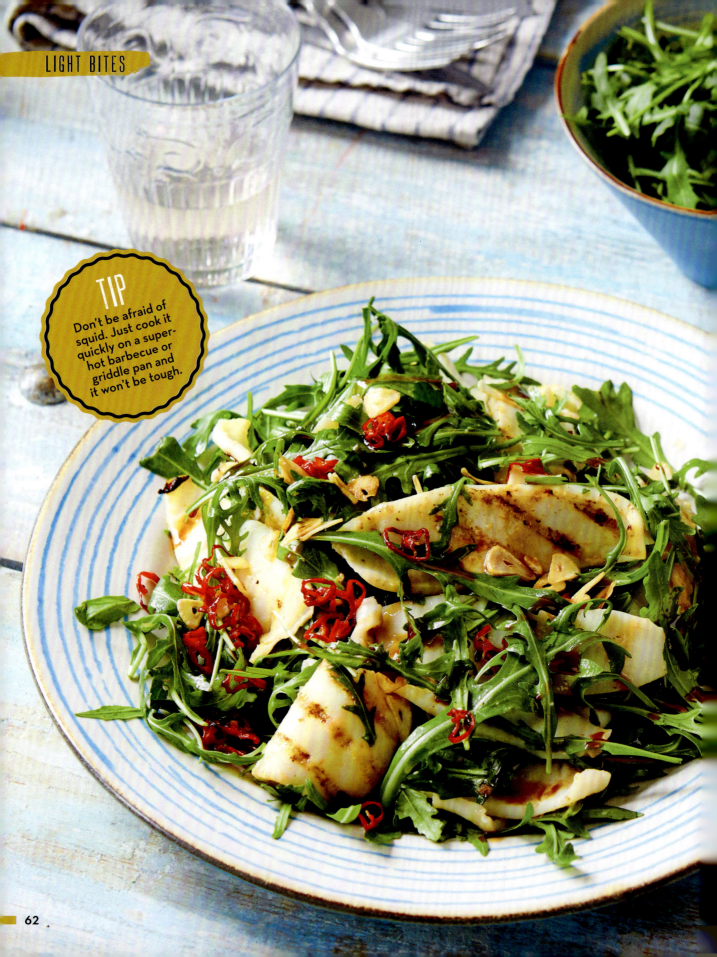

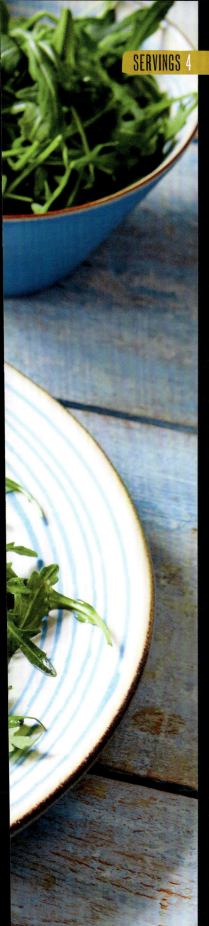

SERVINGS 4 | PREP TIME 5-10 MINS | MARINATING TIME 1 HR - OVERNIGHT | COOK TIME 10 MINS

SQUID SALAD WITH GARLIC AND CHILLI

MASTER THE SIMPLE ART OF COOKING SQUID AND THIS WILL MAKE A TASTY STARTER WHEN ENTERTAINING GUESTS

335 CALORIES

INGREDIENTS

- 800G | 28.2OZ FRESH SQUID, SLICED INTO LARGE PIECES
- 7TBSP OLIVE OIL
- 4 LARGE RED CHILLIES, SLICED
- 6 GARLIC CLOVES, SLICED
- 150G | 5.3OZ ROCKET/ARUGULA
- 2 LEMONS, JUICE ONLY
- SEA SALT

STEP 1 Toss the squid in 2tbsp olive oil with plenty of black pepper. Set aside or you can leave it to marinate overnight in the fridge. Shallow-fry the chillies and garlic in another 2tbsp olive oil until just crispy. Drain on kitchen paper.

STEP 2 Grill the squid on a barbecue until charred on both sides. It literally takes a few mins. Put into a bowl with the remaining 1tbsp olive oil. Toss in the rocket, lemon juice and the chillies and garlic with plenty of sea salt, and serve immediately.

LIGHT BITES

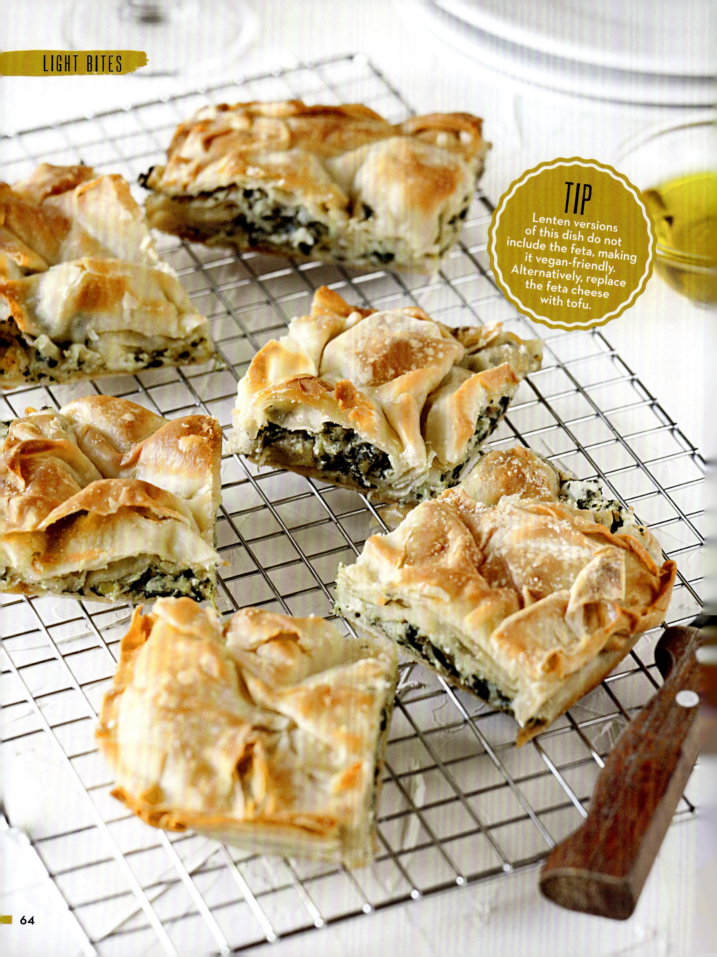

TIP
Lenten versions of this dish do not include the feta, making it vegan-friendly. Alternatively, replace the feta cheese with tofu.

SERVINGS 10-12   PREP TIME 50 MINS   COOK TIME 1 HR

SPANAKOPITA

STUFFED WITH SPINACH AND FETA, THIS FLAKY PASTRY PIE WAS BORN TO BE CONSUMED ON THE STREETS OF ATHENS

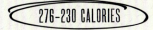
276-230 CALORIES

INGREDIENTS

- 125ML | 4.2FLOZ OLIVE OIL
- 1 ONION, FINELY CHOPPED
- 500G | 17.6OZ FRESH SPINACH
- 2 GARLIC CLOVES
- 200G | 7OZ FETA, CRUMBLED
- 1 HANDFUL FRESH PARSLEY, CHOPPED
- 2 BUNCHES FRESH DILL, CHOPPED (OR 2TBSP DRIED DILL WEED)
- 1 HANDFUL FRESH MINT, CHOPPED (OR 2TBSP DRIED MINT)
- ½ TSP NUTMEG
- FRESHLY GROUND PEPPER
- 3 EGGS, BEATEN
- 1 ROLL SHOP-BOUGHT FILO PASTRY (YOU WILL NEED 12 LEAVES), AT ROOM TEMPERATURE

STEP 1 Preheat the oven to 180°C (160°C fan) | 350°F | gas 4. Brush a 45x30cm | 18x12" rectangular tin with a little olive oil.

STEP 2 Heat 1-2tbsp olive oil in a large pan or pot, and sauté the onion until it is browned and translucent.

STEP 3 Add the spinach and cook until it has wilted. Tip the onion and garlic into a large bowl, and add the feta, herbs, spices and black pepper. Mix together until everything is thoroughly combined.

STEP 4 Add the beaten eggs and 2tbsp olive oil to the spinach filling and mix well until everything is incorporated.

STEP 5 Take one filo sheet out of the packaging and carefully lay it at the bottom of your rectangular pan. Brush it with a little olive oil.

STEP 6 Repeat the previous step with 5 more filo sheets, to make 6 in total.

STEP 7 Spread the spinach and feta mixture evenly within the pan, being careful not to squash it down too much.

STEP 8 Lay a filo sheet on top of the spinach mixture and brush with olive oil. Repeat with 5 more filo sheets, until all your pastry sheets are used up.

STEP 9 Trim the excess filo pastry off and brush the top with olive oil. You can crumble the excess filo pastry and sprinkle it on top of the pie for an extra flaky crust.

STEP 10 Using a knife, score the pastry to mark out 10-12 slices of spanakopita. Be careful not to put the knife all the way through the pastry – only the first couple of layers.

STEP 11 Bake the spanakopita in the oven for about 1 hr, or until golden brown. Leave to cool for about 15 mins, then serve. Alternatively, serve at room temperature – but never cold!

© Getty Images

LIGHT BITES

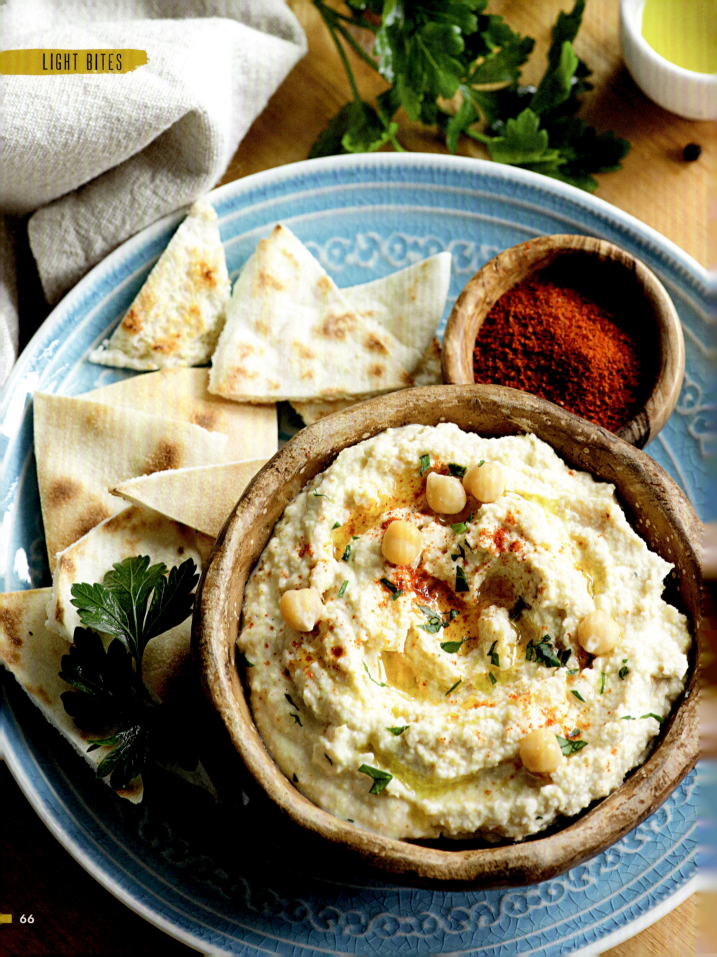

SERVINGS 4   **PREP TIME** 10 MINS   **REST TIME** OVERNIGHT   **COOK TIME** 1 HR

HUMMUS

A DISH SO DELICIOUSLY ICONIC, THE WORLD CONTINUES TO FIGHT OVER ITS ORIGINS

615 CALORIES

INGREDIENTS

- 400G | 14OZ DRIED CHICKPEAS
- 1½ TSP BICARBONATE OF SODA/BAKING SODA
- 5 TBSP (HEAPED) TAHINI (GOOD QUALITY)
- 1 LEMON, JUICED
- 1 GARLIC CLOVE, CRUSHED
- SEA SALT
- EXTRA VIRGIN OLIVE OIL, TO GARNISH
- PAPRIKA, TO GARNISH
- FRESH PARSLEY, TO GARNISH
- 4 SMALL FLATBREADS, TOASTED, TO SERVE

HUMMUS IS SO WIDELY ADORED THAT EVERYONE FROM THE GREEKS TO THE TURKS AND THE NORTH AFRICANS TO THE ARABS CLAIM IT AS THEIR OWN.

STEP 1 Rinse the chickpeas and leave them in a bowl with twice the volume of cold water. Add 1tsp bicarbonate of soda, stir and leave to soak overnight.

STEP 2 Drain the chickpeas and rinse thoroughly under cold water.

STEP 3 Fill a large saucepan with cold water then add the chickpeas and ½tsp bicarbonate of soda. Place on a high heat and bring to the boil, then cover the saucepan and let simmer for about 1 hr. Check it regularly and remove any white foam that forms on top of the water.

STEP 4 To check if the chickpeas are cooked, crush one between your fingers. If it crushes easily and feels smooth, then the chickpeas are ready. Once ready, stir vigorously to loosen the skins and skim away any that come off.

STEP 5 Drain the chickpeas and reserve some of the cooking water. Rinse them well.

STEP 6 Set a few chickpeas aside for a garnish. Place the rest in a food processor and blitz for 1 min. Add the tahini, lemon juice, garlic and salt, then blitz again. Stop to scrape down the sides, and continue blitzing until the mixture becomes creamy and smooth. If the mixture is too thick, add 1tbsp of the chickpea cooking water until the consistency is correct.

STEP 7 Transfer the hummus to a serving bowl, drizzle with extra virgin olive oil, sprinkle with a little paprika and chopped parsley, then top with whole chickpeas. Serve with some toasted flatbreads.

TIP You can use tinned chickpeas instead – simply cook them according to their instructions, then start at step 5.

LIGHT BITES

TIP
The parsley should only be washed in cold water and gently patted dry. Slice it carefully with a sharp knife so that it doesn't get bruised.

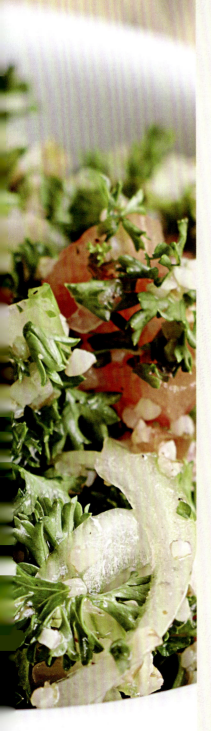

SERVINGS 4 | **PREP TIME 15 MINS** | **COOK TIME 30 MINS**

TABBOULEH

NO LEBANESE FEAST IS COMPLETE WITHOUT THIS ZINGY, PARSLEY-CENTRIC DISH

234 CALORIES

INGREDIENTS

- **75G | 2.6OZ** FINE BULGUR WHEAT
- **4 BUNCHES** FRESH FLAT-LEAF/ITALIAN PARSLEY, LEAVES ONLY, FINELY SLICED
- **1 BUNCH** MINT, FINELY CHOPPED
- **3 MEDIUM** TOMATOES, FINELY CHOPPED
- **1 MEDIUM** ONION, FINELY CHOPPED
- **125ML | 4.2FLOZ** FRESH LEMON JUICE
- **4TBSP** EXTRA VIRGIN OLIVE OIL
- SEA SALT AND FRESHLY GROUND PEPPER

STEP 1 Place the bulgur wheat in a bowl and cover with 2.5cm | 1" of water. Let it sit for 30 mins, until it has doubled in size.

STEP 2 Add the parsley, mint, tomatoes and onion to a mixing large bowl.

STEP 3 Drain the bulgur wheat when it is ready, gently squeezing out any remaining water, and add to the mixing bowl with the herbs and vegetables.

STEP 4 Add the lemon juice, olive oil, salt and pepper, then mix thoroughly. Adjust the seasoning to taste.

Tabbouleh is popular across the Middle East and Europe, but forms an inseparable part of Lebanese culture — the guest of honour at every family dinner and special occasion.

LIGHT BITES

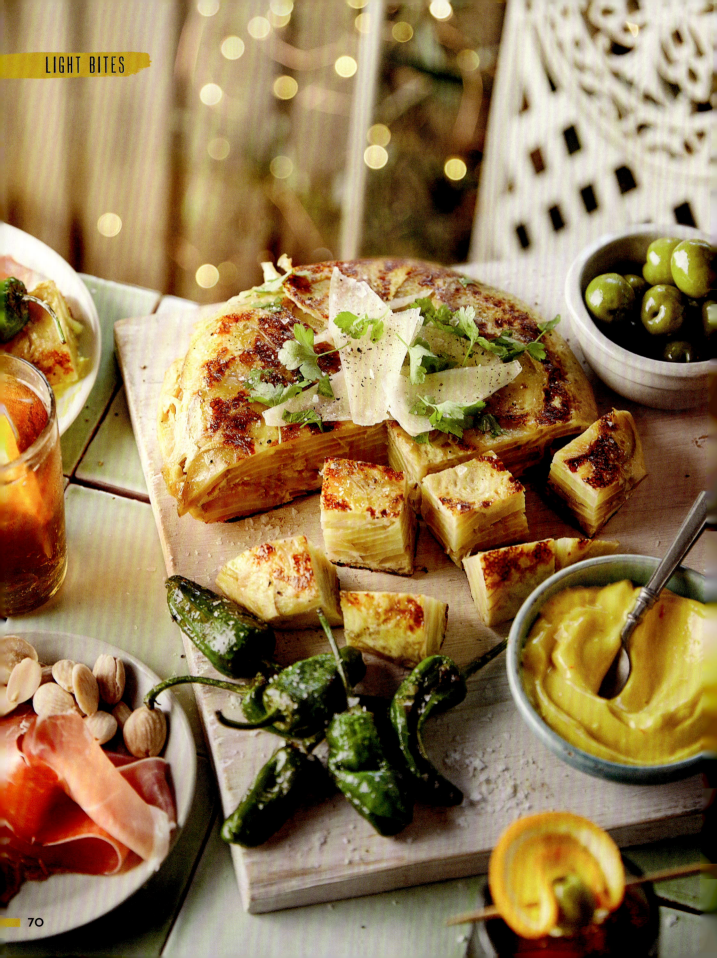

SERVINGS 6   PREP TIME 20 MINS   COOK TIME 40 MINS

SPANISH OMELETTE WITH SAFFRON AIOLI

MAKE THIS CATALONIAN CLASSIC AHEAD OF TIME, THEN WARM IT TO SERVE WITH OTHER TASTY NIBBLES

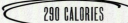

290 CALORIES

INGREDIENTS

FOR THE TORTILLA:
- 30ML | 1FLOZ OLIVE OIL
- 500G | 17.6OZ WAXY POTATOES, UNPEELED, SLICED
- 1 ONION, FINELY SLICED
- 1 SPRIG ROSEMARY
- 1 GARLIC CLOVE, BASHED
- 6 LARGE EGGS
- 2TBSP WHOLE MILK
- FLAKED SEA SALT, SHAVED MANCHEGO AND CHOPPED PARSLEY, TO SERVE

FOR THE AIOLI:
- 1 MEDIUM EGG YOLK
- 1 GARLIC CLOVE, CRUSHED
- SMALL PINCH SAFFRON THREADS
- 1TSP WHITE WINE VINEGAR
- 75ML | 2.5FLOZ OLIVE OIL
- 50ML | 1.7FLOZ VEGETABLE OIL
- JUICE 1/2 LEMON, PLUS WEDGES TO SERVE

STEP 1 For the aioli, combine the egg yolk, garlic, saffron and vinegar in a small food processor with a pinch of salt. Whizz to combine then, with the motor running, slowly pour in the oil, in a thin stream, until thick and creamy. Taste and season with salt and lemon juice.

STEP 2 For the tortilla, heat the oil a 20cm | 8" frying pan over a medium heat. Add the potatoes and fry for 10 mins, stirring until tender but not coloured. Add the onion, rosemary, garlic and some salt, and fry for 10 mins to soften.

STEP 3 In a bowl, beat the eggs with the milk and season. Tip in the potatoes and onion, discarding the rosemary and garlic. Mix well.

STEP 4 Return everything to the pan, reduce the heat to low and cook for 10-15 mins, until it is firm around the edges but a bit runny in the middle.

STEP 5 Remove from the heat, hold a plate over the pan and carefully invert the tortilla. Slide the tortilla off the plate and back into the pan, and cook for 5-10 mins more. Turn out onto a serving board to cool.

STEP 6 Cut the tortilla into cubes, sprinkled with flaked sea salt, shaved Manchego cheese and parsley. Serve with the aioli and any other tasty nibbles.

LIGHT BITES

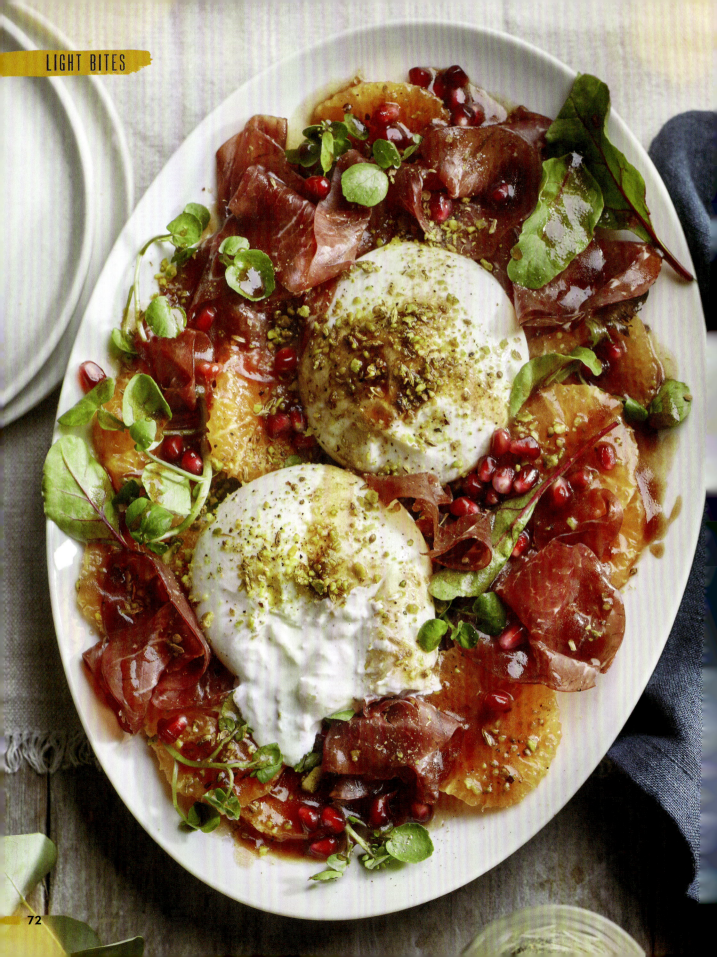

SERVINGS 6 **PREP TIME** 15 MINS **COOK TIME** 5 MINS FOR THE DUKKAH

BURRATA, BRESAOLA AND CLEMENTINE SALAD

THIS SHARING DISH PAIRS ITALIAN FLAVOURS WITH FRAGRANT EGYPTIAN DUKKAH

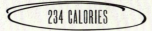
234 CALORIES

INGREDIENTS

3 CLEMENTINES, PEELED AND SLICED
60G | 2OZ BAG BABY SALAD LEAVES
70G | 2.5OZ PACK BRESAOLA
2X 150G | 5OZ BURRATA
POMEGRANATE SEEDS, TO SERVE

FOR THE DUKKAH:
2TBSP PISTACHIOS
1TSP FENNEL SEEDS
1/2TSP CORIANDER SEEDS
1/2TSP FLAKY SEA SALT

FOR THE DRESSING:
3TBSP EXTRA VIRGIN OLIVE OIL
2TSP POMEGRANATE MOLASSES
1TSP BALSAMIC VINEGAR
(OR USE RED WINE VINEGAR)
JUICE 1/2 CLEMENTINE

STEP 1 For the dukkah, in a small pan, toast the pistachios, then remove to a pestle and mortar. Add the seeds to the pan and toast until fragrant, then add to the pestle and mortar with the salt and a few grinds of black pepper. Grind to make a crumb.

STEP 2 Mix together the dressing ingredients, then season with salt and pepper.

STEP 3 Arrange the clementine slices, salad and bresaola on a platter, then nestle the burrata on the top. Sprinkle with the dukkah and drizzle over the dressing, then scatter with pomegranate seeds.

YOU CAN USE ANY LEFTOVER DUKKAH TO SPRINKLE OVER ROASTED VEG SUCH AS CARROTS, IF THIS IS FOLLOWED BY A MAIN MEAL.

LIGHT BITES

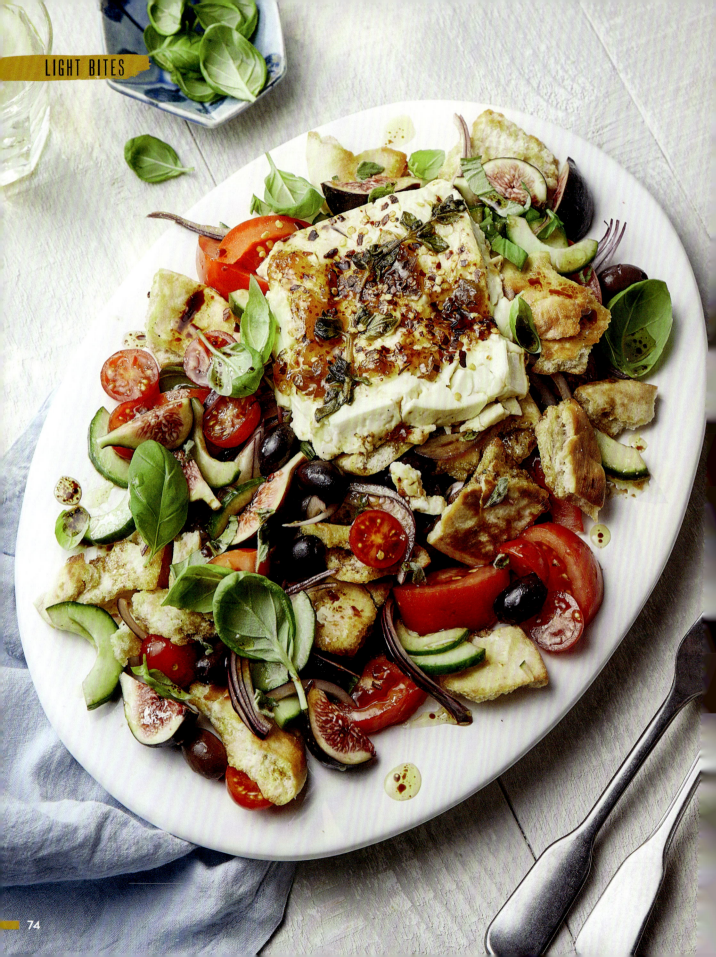

SERVINGS 4   PREP TIME 15 MINS   COOK TIME 20 MINS

BAKED FETA GREEK SALAD WITH FIGS

JAMMY, SALTY FETA GIVES SWEETNESS AND DEPTH TO THIS UPDATED CLASSIC

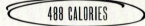
488 CALORIES

INGREDIENTS

- 250G | 9OZ FETA
- 1TBSP FIG CONSERVE
- 2TBSP EXTRA VIRGIN OLIVE OIL
- 1/2TSP CHILLI FLAKES
- SPRIGS OF FRESH OREGANO OR 1TSP OREGANO
- 400G | 14OZ MIXED TOMATOES, CHOPPED
- 1/2 CUCUMBER, DESEEDED AND SLICED INTO HALF-MOONS
- 1/2 RED ONION, THINLY SLICED
- SMALL BUNCH BASIL, FINELY CHOPPED, PLUS EXTRA TO SERVE
- 2-4 PITTA BREADS, ROUGHLY TORN
- 150G | 5OZ KALAMATA OLIVES, SLICED IN HALF
- 2-4 FIGS, QUARTERED

FOR THE DRESSING:
- 3TBSP EXTRA VIRGIN OLIVE OIL
- 1TBSP BALSAMIC VINEGAR

STEP 1 Heat the oven 200°C (180°C fan) | 400°F | gas 6. Line a medium size baking tray with foil and put the whole feta block in the middle. Spread over the fig conserve, 1tbsp oil, the chilli flakes and oregano. Roast for 10-15 mins until starting to turn golden.

STEP 2 Meanwhile, chop the tomatoes into various shapes and add to a large bowl with the cucumber, onion and basil. Season and mix through the dressing.

STEP 3 Toss the torn pitta bread in a bowl with the remaining oil and season well. After 8-10 mins add the pitta and half the olives to the baking tray and roast for another 6-7 mins. Add the quartered figs for the final few mins, until they start to become jammy.

STEP 4 To serve, add the tomatoes and cucumber to a platter with the pittas, olives, figs and feta. Top with extra basil and pepper.

Serve the baked feta as a light lunch or as a fancy side with grilled lamb, chicken or steak.

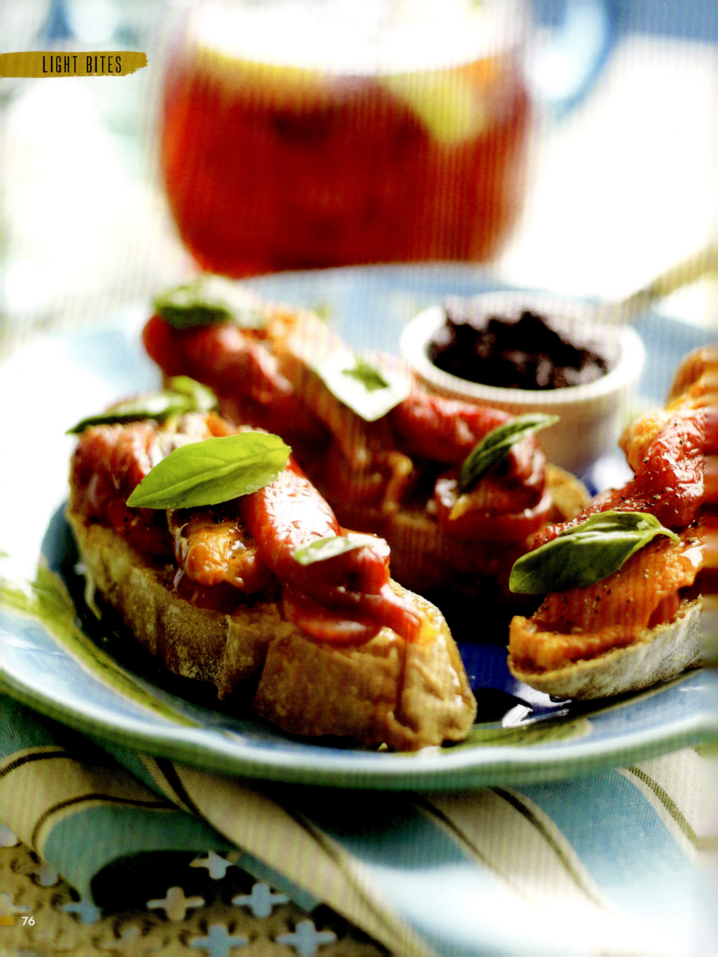
LIGHT BITES

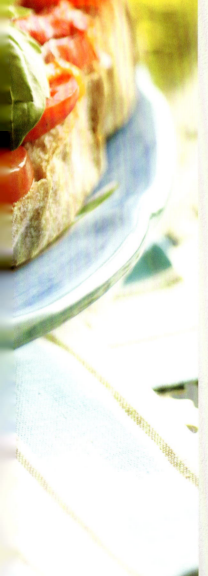

SERVINGS 8 **PREP TIME** 15 MINS **COOK TIME** 50 MINS

ROASTED PEPPER AND GARLIC BRUSCHETTA

THE CLASSIC ITALIAN BRUSCHETTA WITH A SPANISH TWIST

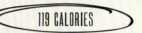

119 CALORIES

INGREDIENTS

- 1 BULB OF GARLIC
- 3 RED OR YELLOW BELL PEPPERS
- 8 SLICES CIABATTA, TOASTED
- 16 CHERRY TOMATOES, SLICED
- BASIL LEAVES
- OLIVE OIL, TO DRIZZLE
- BLACK OLIVE TAPENADE, TO SERVE

STEP 1 Heat the oven to 200°C (180°C fan) | 400°F | gas 6. Wrap the bulb of garlic in foil and put in a roasting tin with the peppers. Cook for 40 mins, until the peppers are soft and slightly blackened.

STEP 2 Put the peppers in a bowl, cover with cling film and leave to steam for 10 mins.

STEP 3 Once cool enough to handle, peel away the skins from the peppers, and the tops and seeds. Cut into strips and set aside.

STEP 4 Remove the garlic from the foil and squeeze the cloves out from their skins. Spread one onto each slice of ciabatta, then put tomato slices on top, followed by strips of pepper, basil leaves, seasoning and a drizzle of olive oil. Serve with the tapenade on the side to dip into.

LIGHT BITES

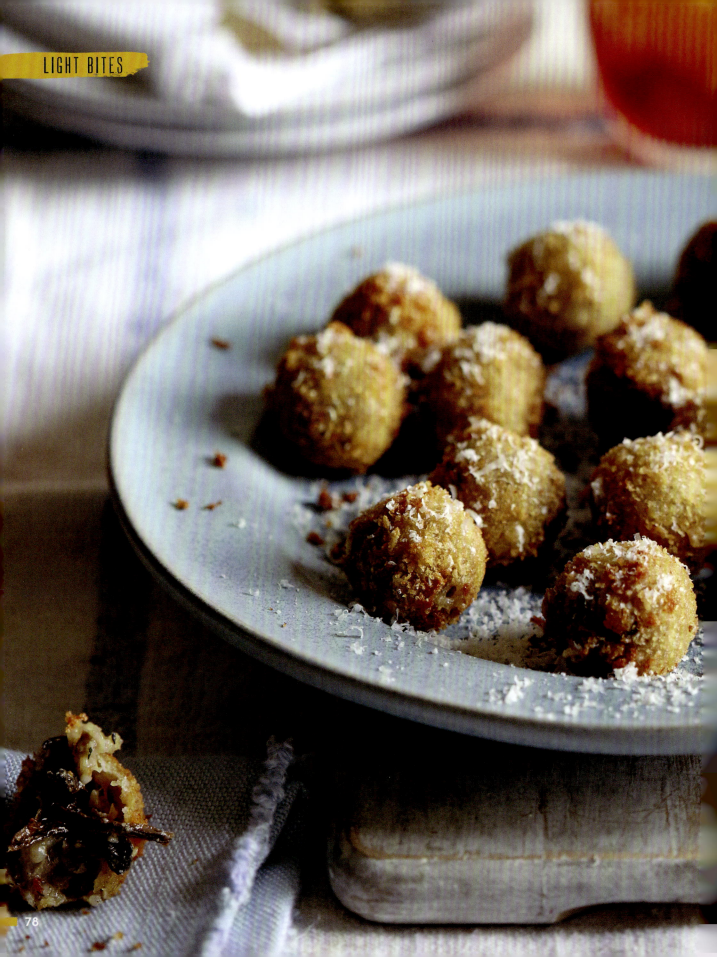

MAKES 20 | **PREP TIME 1 HR** | **COOK TIME 1 HR 15 MINS**

LAMB ARANCINI

THIS SICILIAN STREET FOOD MAKES A TASTY STARTER OR SNACK

255 CALORIES

INGREDIENTS

2TBSP OLIVE OIL
100G | 3.5OZ CARROTS, VERY FINELY DICED
100G | 3.5OZ ONION, VERY FINELY DICED
100G | 3.5OZ CELERY, VERY FINELY DICED
1 GARLIC CLOVE, CRUSHED
300G | 10.6OZ LAMB MINCE
1TSP TOMATO PURÉE /PASTE
300G | 10.6OZ RISOTTO RICE
375ML | 12.7FLOZ DRY WHITE WINE
1L | 2PT HOT LAMB STOCK
2X 125G | 4.4OZ BALLS MOZZARELLA, DICED
200G | 7OZ EMMENTAL, GRATED

FOR THE CRUST:
100G | 3.5OZ FLOUR
2 EGGS, BEATEN
200G | 7OZ PANKO BREADCRUMBS
VEGETABLE OR GROUNDNUT OIL, FOR DEEP-FRYING

STEP 1 Heat the olive oil in a large pan and sauté the carrots, onion, celery and garlic for 5 mins, until soft but with no colour.

STEP 2 Add the lamb mince and brown just to remove the redness. Spoon in the tomato purée and cook for 3 mins, then stir in the rice and deglaze the pan with the wine. Start to add the stock and cook the risotto for 20 mins, gradually adding the hot stock a ladle at a time.

STEP 3 Once the rice is al dente (just cooked), allow it to cool on a large tray so it's flat. When cooled, mix the cooked rice with the diced mozzarella and grated Emmental. Check the seasoning and add more salt and pepper if necessary.

STEP 4 Roll into 20 balls and allow to set in the fridge (at least 1 hr). When ready, dip into the flour, then the beaten egg and the panko breadcrumbs. In a deep fat fryer or suitable pan, heat the oil to 180°C | 350°F and fry the arancini in batches until golden brown.

LIGHT BITES

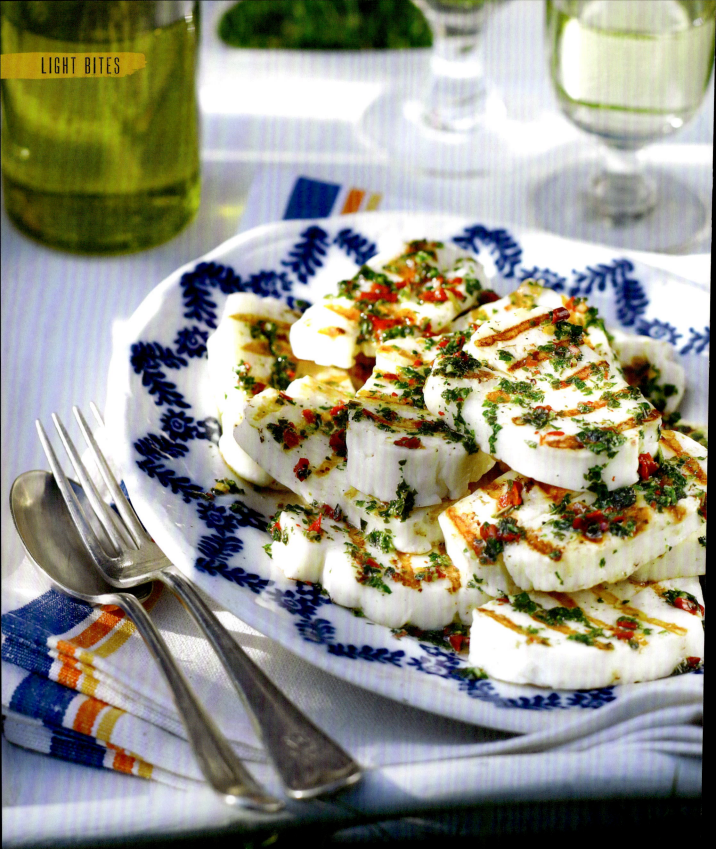

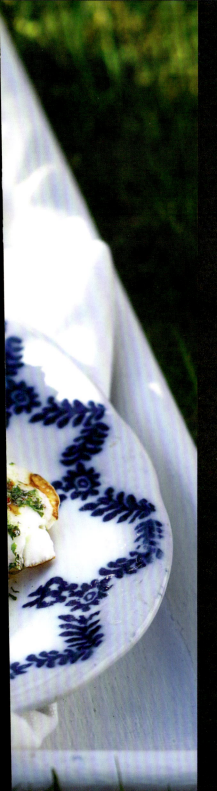

SERVINGS 6-8 PREP TIME 5 MINS COOK TIME 5 MINS

HALLOUMI WITH A CHILLI KICK

HALLOUMI IS THE PERFECT CHEESE FOR THE BARBECUE – THE FIRM TEXTURE MEANS IT SOFTENS SLIGHTLY BUT STILL KEEPS ITS SHAPE WHEN COOKED

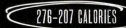

276-207 CALORIES

INGREDIENTS

1TBSP OLIVE OIL
1TSP VERY LAZY CHOPPED RED CHILLIES
2TBSP LEMON JUICE
2TSP FROZEN MINT
500G | 17.6OZ HALLOUMI, CUT INTO 1.5CM | 0.6" SLICES

STEP 1 To make the sauce, mix the oil, chillies, lemon juice and mint together in a jug with some freshly ground black pepper.

STEP 2 Cook the halloumi on the barbecue for 1-2 mins each side until evenly charred. Transfer to a serving platter and drizzle over the chilli sauce.

LIGHT BITES

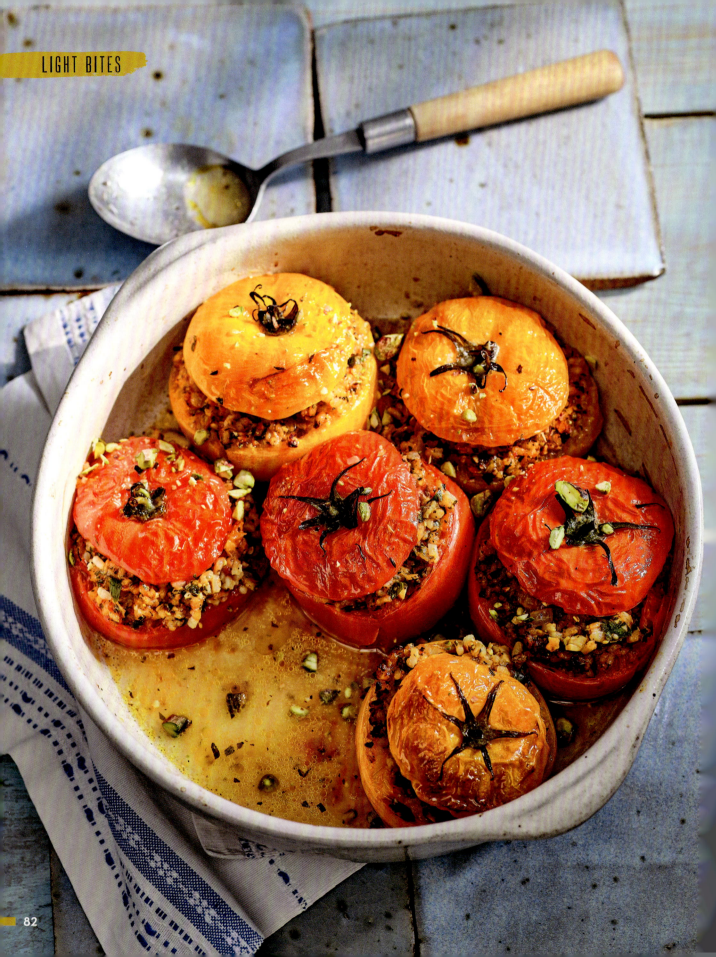

SERVINGS 6-8   PREP TIME 5 MINS   COOK TIME 50 MINS

BAKED STUFFED TOMATOES WITH HARISSA RICE

THIS FILLING VEGGIE DISH IS FULL OF FLAVOUR. STUFFED AND BAKED VEGETABLE DISHES ARE EATEN ACROSS THE EASTERN MEDITERRANEAN AND MAKE IDEAL INDIVIDUAL SERVINGS AS PART OF A SHARING MENU

180-135 CALORIES

INGREDIENTS

- **300ML | 10FLOZ** VEGETABLE STOCK
- **100G | 3.5OZ** SHORT-GRAIN RICE, SUCH AS PAELLA OR ARBORIO RICE
- AROUND **2TBSP** OLIVE OIL
- **1** ONION, FINELY CHOPPED
- **2** FAT GARLIC CLOVES, CRUSHED
- **1TSP** DRIED MINT
- **1/2TSP** MIXED SPICE
- **6** MEDIUM OR **8** SMALL BEEF TOMATOES
- **1TBSP** ROSE HARISSA
- **4TBSP** PISTACHIOS, CHOPPED
- LARGE HANDFUL EACH FRESH PARSLEY, MINT AND OREGANO, ROUGHLY CHOPPED
- **75ML | 2.5FLOZ** DRY WHITE WINE
- **50G | 1.0OZ** BUTTER, CUBED (OR USE OIL IF MAKING A VEGAN/DAIRY-FREE VERSION)

STEP 1 Heat the oven to 190°C (190°C fan) | 375°F | gas 5. In a pan, bring the stock to the boil, then tip in the rice, a glug of oil, salt and ground black pepper. Bring back up to a fast simmer, then turn down the heat and simmer gently until tender and all the liquid is absorbed. (Top up with a little more boiling water if needed). Take off the heat.

STEP 2 Heat a glug of olive oil in a frying pan and cook the onion for 5 mins until beginning to soften. Add the garlic, cook for 2 mins, then stir in the mint and mixed spice.

STEP 3 Cut a 2cm | 0.8" slice off the top of each beef tomato and put them aside. Use a teaspoon to scoop out the pulp inside. Put the pulp in a sieve, set over a bowl, to drain away the excess water. Roughly chop the tomato flesh left in the sieve, then add to the onion and garlic. Increase the heat and cook until the mixture has reduced and thickened – about 5-10 mins.

STEP 4 Stir in the rose harissa, and most of the pistachios and herbs. Add the cooked grains and stir again until combined.

STEP 5 Put the hollowed-out beef tomatoes in a lightly oiled baking dish, then fill with the rice mixture. Put the reserved tomato tops back on, then pour over the wine and dot the butter over the tomatoes. Bake for 25-30 mins, basting halfway through with the cooking juices, until the tomatoes are tender. Garnish with the remaining nuts and herbs. Serve hot or at room temperature, if liked.

LIGHT BITES

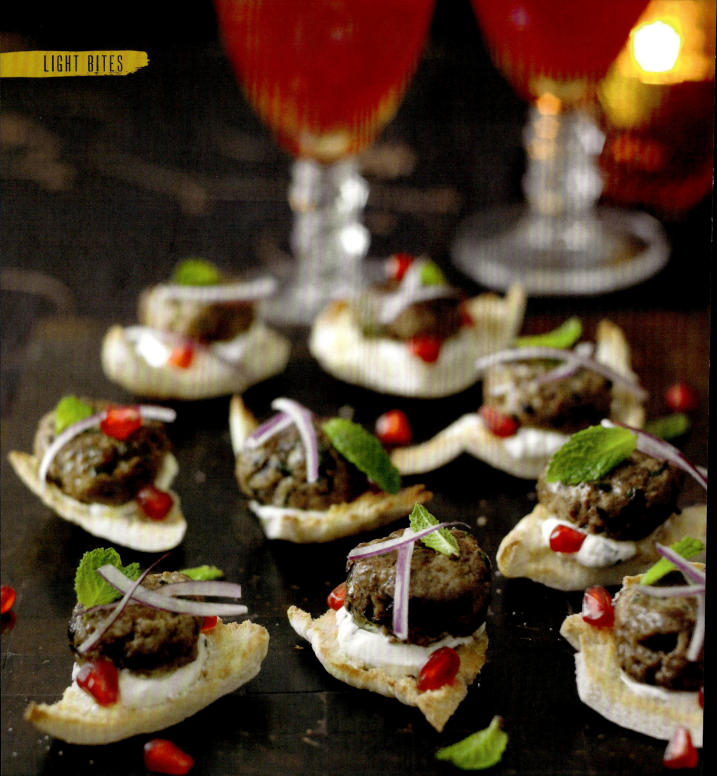

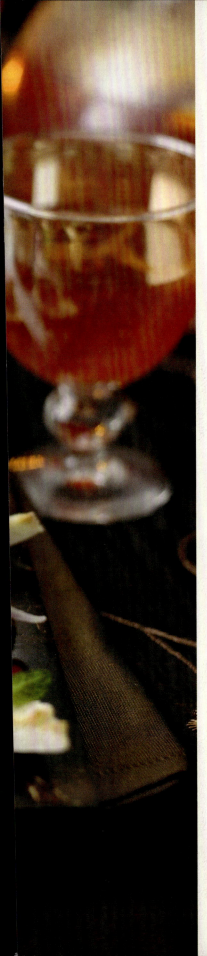

MAKES 18   PREP TIME 25 MINS   COOK TIME 5 MINS

LAMB PITTA BITES

SPICE THINGS UP WITH THESE PARCELS OF LAMB, A BLEND OF GREEK AND MOROCCAN FLAVOURS

148 CALORIES

INGREDIENTS

250G | 8.8OZ MINCED LAMB
4TSP RAS EL HANOUT
4TBSP CHOPPED FRESH MINT, PLUS BABY MINT LEAVES FOR GARNISH
150G | 5.3OZ PLAIN GREEK YOGHURT
3 PITTA BREADS
1/2TBSP SUNFLOWER OR OLIVE OIL
1 SMALL RED ONION, SLICED, MIXED WITH
1TBSP LEMON JUICE
SEEDS OF 1/2 POMEGRANATE

STEP 1 Mix together the lamb, ras el hanout, half the mint and a pinch of salt. Using lightly oiled hands, shape the mixture into 18 small patties, transfer to a plate, cover and chill until ready to cook. Stir the remaining mint into the yoghurt and season.

STEP 2 Heat the grill to high. Split each pitta bread in half horizontally. Cut each half into 3 triangles and put on a baking tray. Grill for 1-2 mins on one side until golden and crisp.

STEP 3 When ready to serve, heat the oil in a non-stick frying pan. Add the lamb patties and fry for 2 mins on each side until cooked through.

STEP 4 Spoon a dollop of the yoghurt mixture onto each pitta triangle, then add a lamb patty and some onion. Garnish with the baby mint leaves and pomegranate.

LIGHT BITES

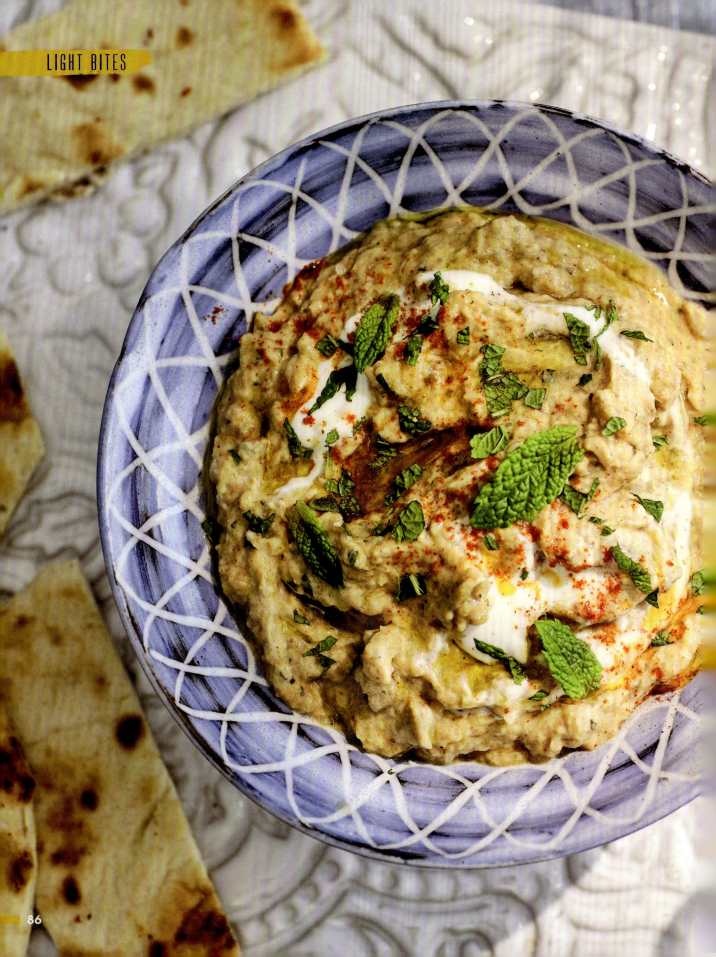

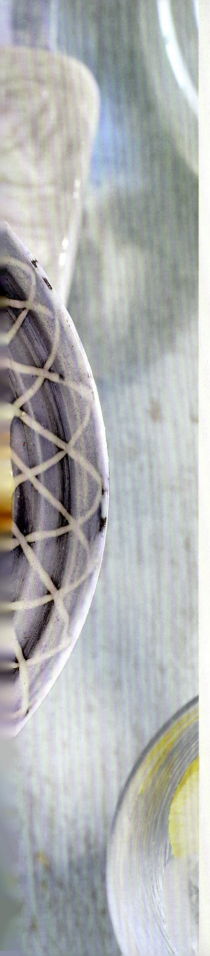

SERVINGS 6-8 | **PREP TIME 10 MINS, PLUS COOLING** | **COOK TIME 30 MINS**

BABA GANOUSH

INSPIRED BY LEBANESE BABA GANOUSH, OUR RECIPE USES YOGHURT FOR AN EXTRA-CREAMY TEXTURE

61-46 CALORIES

INGREDIENTS

- 2 LARGE AUBERGINES/EGGPLANTS
- 1 TSP SMOKED PAPRIKA, PLUS EXTRA FOR SPRINKLING
- 1 TBSP TAHINI
- 1/2 TSP DRIED MINT
- 2 GARLIC CLOVES, CRUSHED
- 4 TBSP NATURAL YOGHURT, PLUS EXTRA TO SERVE
- 1 TBSP EXTRA VIRGIN OLIVE OIL
- FRESH MINT LEAVES, TO SERVE

STEP 1 Heat the grill and prick each aubergine with a fork. Grill on a foil-lined grilled tray, turning regularly for 20-30 mins, until charred all over. Remove and set aside to cool.

STEP 2 Once cool enough to handle, peel off the aubergine skin and discard, then roughly chop the flesh and put it in a sieve to drain off excess moisture.

STEP 3 Mix the paprika, tahini, mint, garlic and most of the yoghurt in a bowl, mash in the aubergine and season to taste.

STEP 4 Spoon into a serving bowl. Swirl in the extra yoghurt, and olive oil. Sprinkle with paprika and fresh mint leaves.

LIGHT BITES

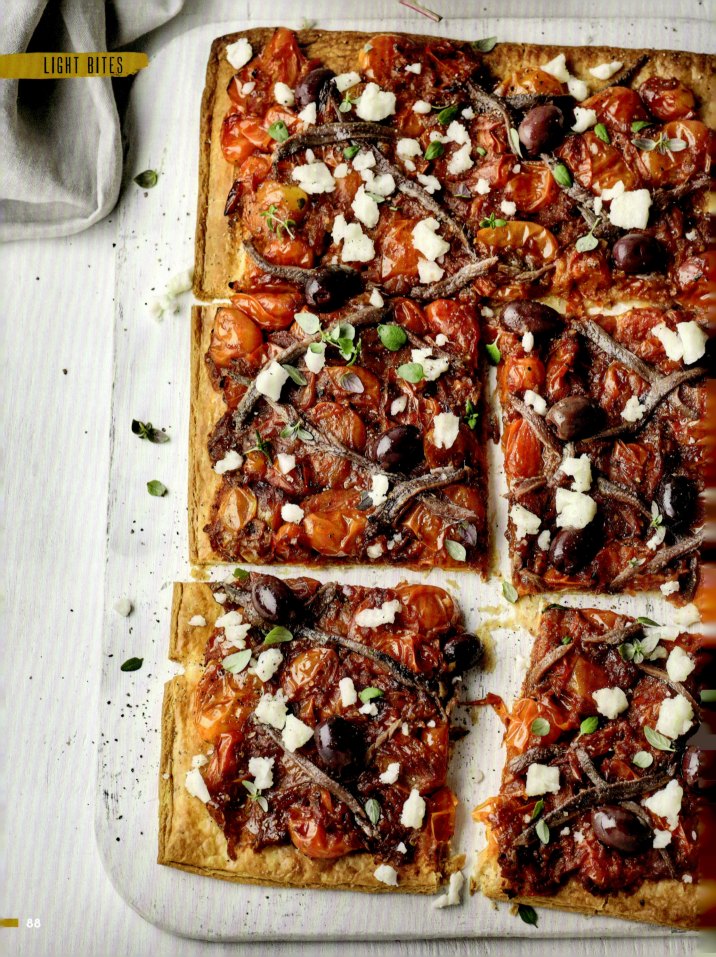

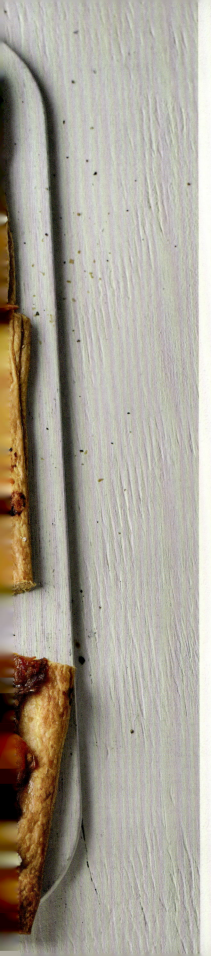

SERVINGS 6   PREP TIME 25 MINS   COOK TIME 22 MINS

PISSALADIÈRE

OUR TAKE ON THE CLASSIC FRENCH TART HITS THE SPOT – IT'S SUMMER IN A SLICE!

270 CALORIES

INGREDIENTS

- 320G | 11.3 PACK READY-ROLLED LIGHT PUFF PASTRY
- 30G | 1OZ TIN ANCHOVY FILLETS IN OIL
- 2 RED ONIONS, DICED
- 800G | 28.2OZ RIPE PLUM TOMATOES, ROUGHLY CHOPPED
- 2 GARLIC CLOVES, CRUSHED
- 5 SPRIGS THYME, LEAVES PICKED
- 1 BAY LEAF
- 1/2TSP GROUND NUTMEG
- 50G | 1.8OZ PITTED BLACK OLIVES
- 10G | 0.4OZ CRUMBLY GOAT'S CHEESE
- GREEN SALAD, TO SERVE

STEP 1 Heat the oven to 220°C (200°C fan) | 425°F | gas 6. Unroll the pastry sheet on its baking paper and put it on an oven tray. Prick over with a fork, then cover with another sheet of baking paper and lay another baking tray over it. Cook for 15 mins with the tray on top.

STEP 2 Meanwhile, heat 1tbsp of the oil from the tin of anchovies in a large shallow pan, and sweat the onions until golden and translucent. Add the tomatoes, garlic, thyme, bay leaf, nutmeg and 3 of the anchovies. Season and cook for 10-15 mins until broken down.

STEP 3 Remove the pastry from the oven; spread over the tomato mix (remove the bay leaf). Return to the oven for a further 20 mins.

STEP 4 As the tart cooks, slice the remaining anchovies in half lengthways. Arrange these in a lattice pattern on the tart, placing an olive into the centre of each diamond. Scatter over the cheese and return to the oven for a further 2 mins. Serve warm with a salad on the side.

LIGHT BITES

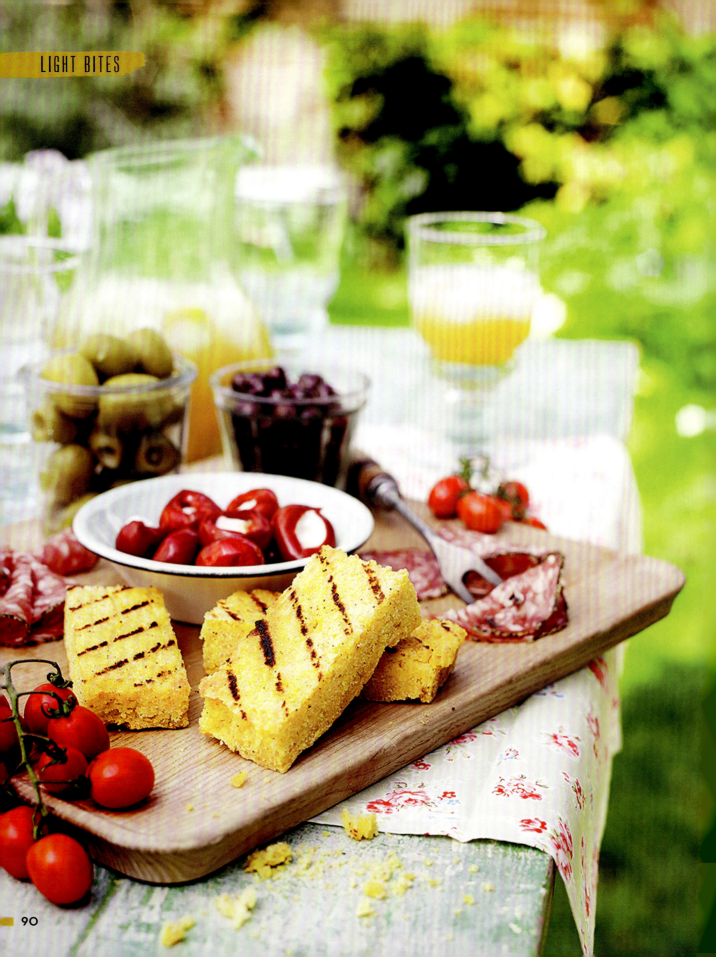

SERVINGS 12 SLICES | PREP TIME 15 MINS | COOK TIME 20 MINS

POLENTA BREAD WITH ANTIPASTI

BECAUSE OF THE CORNMEAL, THIS HAS QUITE A UNIQUE TEXTURE AND IS QUICKER TO MAKE THAN NORMAL BREAD

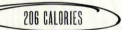

206 CALORIES

INGREDIENTS

- 225G | 7.9OZ POLENTA (CORNMEAL)
- 225G | 7.9OZ PLAIN FLOUR
- 50G | 1.8OZ CASTER SUGAR
- 1 TBSP BAKING POWDER
- 225ML | 7.6FLOZ BUTTERMILK
- 1 LARGE EGG, BEATEN
- 60G (2.1OZ) BUTTER, MELTED
- OLIVE OIL, TO DRIZZLE

YOU WILL NEED:
A 30X20CM | 11.8X7.9" BROWNIE TIN, OILED AND LINED WITH BAKING PAPER

STEP 1 Heat the oven to 220°C (200°C fan) | 425°F | gas 6. In a large bowl mix together the polenta, flour, sugar, baking powder and 1/2tsp salt. Add the buttermilk and beaten egg and stir well. Add the melted butter and combine. Pour into the baking tin and bake for 20 mins. Allow to cool in the tin for 20 mins then turn out onto a wire rack. Once cold you can tightly wrap it until you are ready to grill it or put into the freezer.

STEP 2 Cut the loaf into long, chunky slices, drizzle with olive oil and grill. Serve with a selection of antipasti. We had mini stuffed peppers, salami and olives.

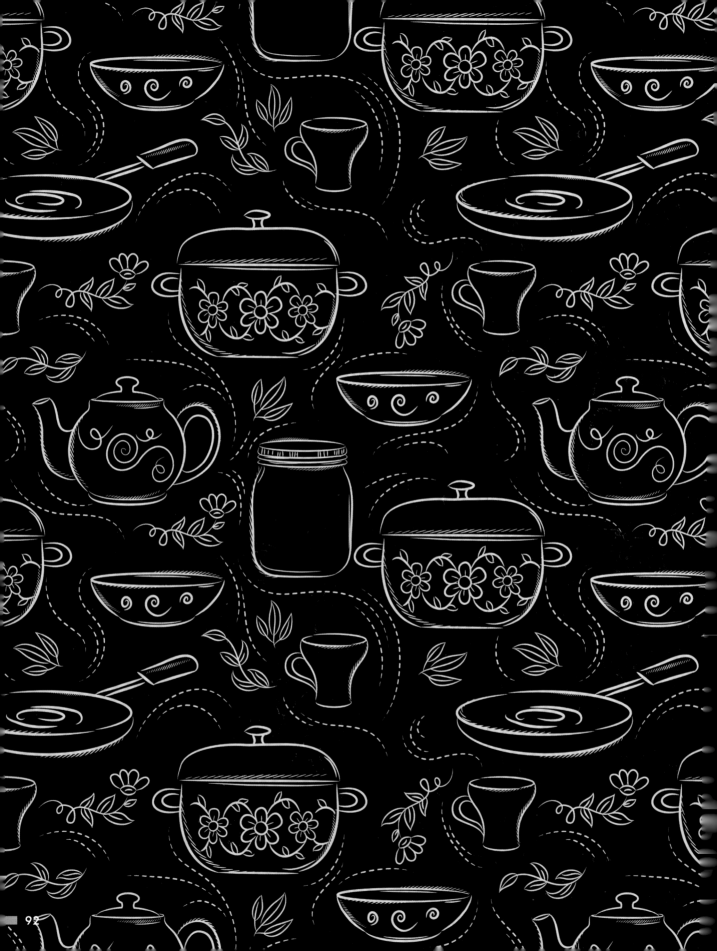

MAIN MEALS

Spanish chicken bake 95
White bean & tomato salad 97
Stuffed mackerel 99
Moussaka 101
Mediterranean lamb with feta stuffing 103
Summer ratatouille.. 105
Chicken stuffed with basil................................. 107
Timballo Siciliano 109
Fisherman's sea bream with aioli 111
Vegetarian lasagne 113
Portuguese-style beef skewers
with French beans.. 115
Tomato and couscous salad 117
Provençal fish traybake......................................119
Mediterranean vegetable calzone...................121
Lamb cutlets with pea and mint purée 123
Mediterranean veg rolls..................................... 125
Catalan fish stew.. 127
Risotto al funghi 129
Salmon & spaghetti Bolognese 131
Couscous and chickpea salad...........................133
Paella.. 135
Mediterranean sea bass bake 137
Mussels with chorizo 139
Med-style chicken with basil and olives 141
Chicken shawarma 143
Greek roast chicken gyros 145
Chicken parmigiana... 147
Veal steak with polenta 149
Pork chops with orzo..151
Pork Milanese with saffron risotto 153
Salmon parcels.. 155
Portuguese sardines.. 157
Fried squid.. 159
Falafel halloumi skewers....................................161

MAIN MEALS

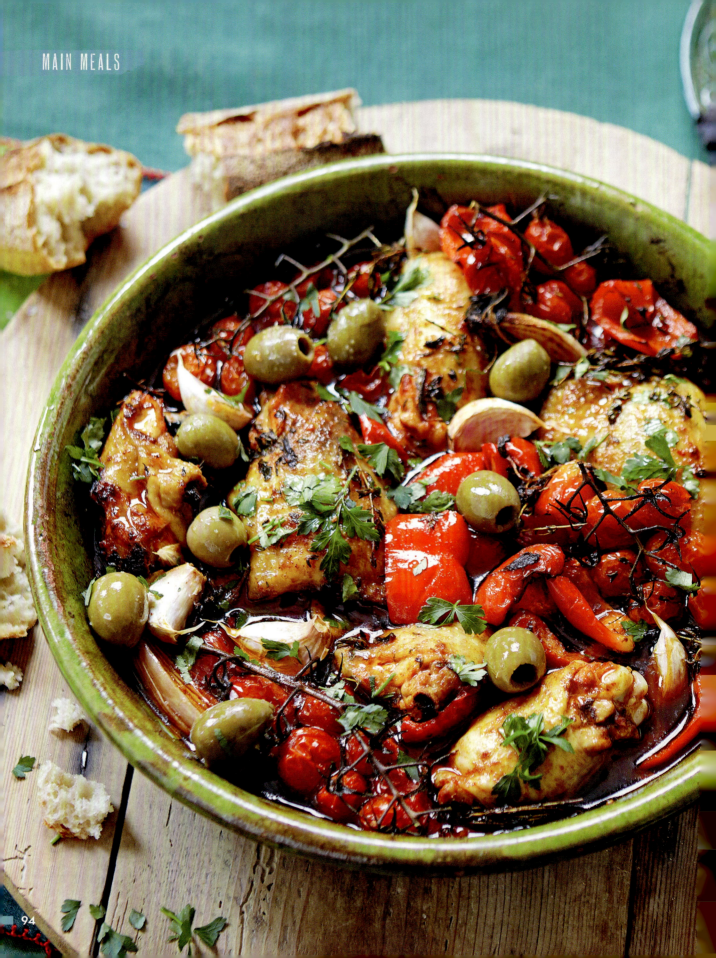

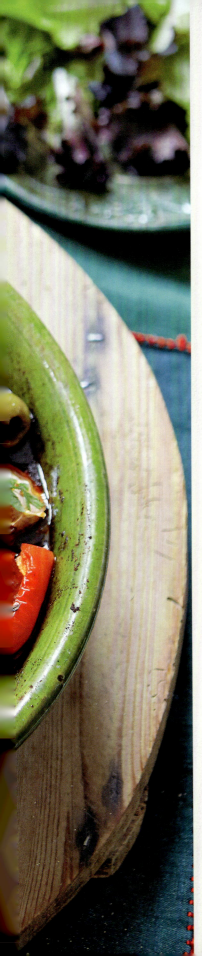

SERVINGS 4 | **PREP TIME 15 MINS** | **COOK TIME 1 HR 15 MINS**

SPANISH CHICKEN BAKE

PACKED FULL OF FLAVOUR, THIS MOUTH-WATERING DISH IS WONDERFULLY SIMPLE TO MAKE

375 CALORIES

INGREDIENTS

- 250G | 8.8OZ CHERRY TOMATOES
- 2 SHALLOTS, SLICED INTO WEDGES
- 2 RED BELL PEPPERS, ROUGHLY CHOPPED
- 8 CHICKEN THIGHS
- 1 BUNCH EACH OF THYME AND OREGANO
- 2TBSP SWEET SMOKED PAPRIKA
- 4TBSP OLIVE OIL
- 1 GLASS WHITE WINE
- 6 GARLIC CLOVES, UNPEELED
- 100G | 3.5OZ PITTED GREEN OLIVES
- CRUSTY BREAD, TO SERVE

STEP 1 Preheat the oven to 180°C (160°C fan) | 350°F | gas 4. Toss the tomatoes, shallots, peppers, chicken, thyme and oregano with the paprika and olive oil in a large roasting tin.

STEP 2 Pour over the wine and roast for 45 mins. Add the garlic and cook for another 30 mins until the chicken is cooked through. Top with olives and serve with bread.

MAIN MEALS

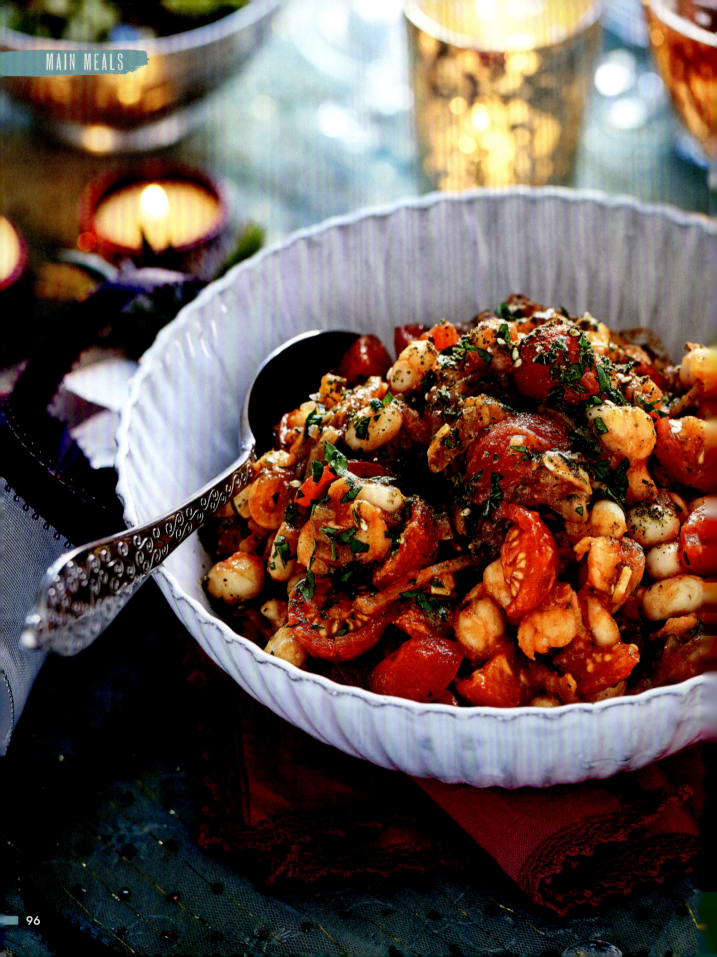

SERVINGS 8   **PREP TIME** 5-10 MINS   **REST TIME** 1 HR   **COOK TIME** 15 MINS

WHITE BEAN & TOMATO SALAD

THIS EGYPTIAN DISH IS A DELICIOUS WAY TO ENJOY PROTEIN-PACKED BEANS

132 CALORIES

INGREDIENTS

- **3TBSP** OLIVE OIL
- **2** LARGE ONIONS, SLICED
- **2** GARLIC CLOVES, CRUSHED
- **70G | 2.5OZ** TOMATO PURÉE/PASTE
- **1** LEMON, JUICE ONLY
- **660G | 23.3OZ** TINNED HARICOT/NAVY BEANS, DRAINED AND RINSED (SEE TIP)
- **250G | 8.8OZ** CHERRY TOMATOES, QUARTERED
- **5TBSP** CHOPPED FLAT-LEAF/ITALIAN PARSLEY
- **1TBSP** ZA'ATAR

STEP 1 Heat 1tbsp oil in a pan. Gently cook the onions for 10 mins then add the garlic and stir through for a few mins. Add 150ml | 5floz water and the tomato purée. Stir well then put into a bowl, covered, to cool completely.

STEP 2 Stir the remaining olive oil and the lemon juice into the onions together with the beans. Add the tomatoes and parsley. Check the seasoning and adjust to taste, then sprinkle over the za'atar.

TIP

You can alternatively use dried beans prepared as per the packet instructions, or follow steps 1-5 on page 67, simmering until tender.

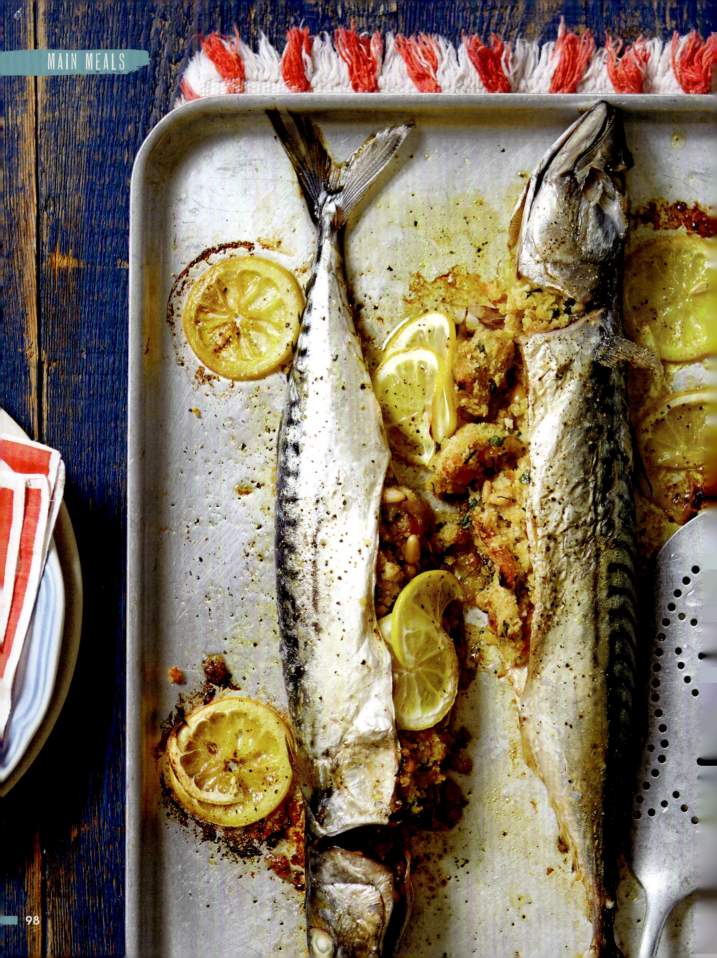

MAIN MEALS

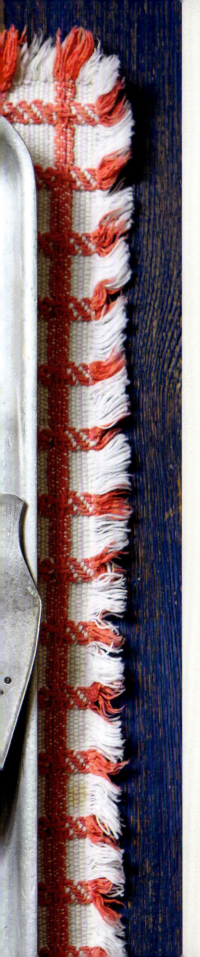

SERVINGS 8 PREP TIME 15-20 MINS COOK TIME 20 MINS

STUFFED MACKEREL

THIS IS A SIMPLE AND TASTY WAY TO ENJOY OILY FISH, WHICH ARE AN IMPORTANT PART OF THE MEDITERRANEAN DIET

352 CALORIES

INGREDIENTS

- 100G | 3.5OZ FRESH BREADCRUMBS
- 40G | 1.4OZ DRIED APRICOTS, ROUGHLY CHOPPED
- 2 TBSP TOASTED PINE NUTS
- 2 LEMONS, 1 ZESTED AND JUICED, ½ SLICED AND ½ CUT INTO WEDGES TO SERVE
- 3 TBSP FLAT-LEAF/ITALIAN PARSLEY, CHOPPED
- 4 TBSP OLIVE OIL
- 2 WHOLE MACKEREL, GUTTED

STEP 1 Preheat the oven to 200°C (180°C fan) | 400°F | gas 6. Combine the breadcrumbs, apricots, pine nuts, lemon zest and juice, parsley and half the oil with plenty of seasoning.

STEP 2 Open up the mackerel, stuff the mixture inside and drizzle the remaining oil on the outside, with plenty of seasoning. Spread a few lemon slices over the top of the fish and tuck a few into the cavity.

STEP 3 Put the fish on a baking tray and cook for 20 mins, until just cooked through.

STEP 4 To serve, place the fish on a platter with lemon wedges.

TIP
Leaving the fish whole and serving on a platter like this makes a great impact when you're entertaining.

MAIN MEALS

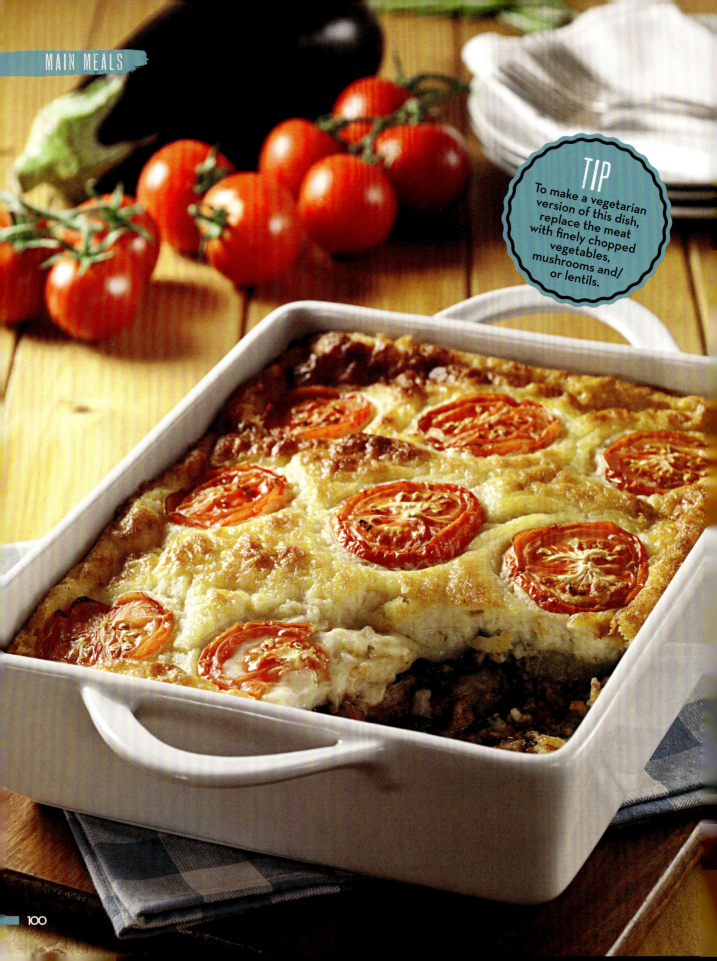

TIP
To make a vegetarian version of this dish, replace the meat with finely chopped vegetables, mushrooms and/or lentils.

MOUSSAKA

RICH LAYERS OF VEGETABLES, MEAT AND CREAMY WHITE SAUCE MAKE UP GREECE'S BEST-LOVED DISH

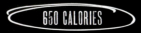

650 CALORIES

SERVINGS 8 — **PREP TIME 45 MINS** — **COOK TIME 45 MINS - 1 HR**

STEP 1 Preheat the oven to 180°C (160°C fan) | 350°F | gas 4. Heat 1-2tbsp of oil in a frying pan over a high heat and fry the aubergine and courgette slices until soft. Drain on some kitchen paper.

STEP 2 To start the meat sauce, warm another 1-2tbsp of oil in a deep saucepan over a medium heat. Fry the onion until soft. Add the garlic and cook for another 2 mins, before adding the thyme and sugar, then continue to fry until everything has caramelised.

STEP 3 Add the lamb mince and tomato purée. Break up any big chunks of mince, and cook until golden brown. Add the red wine (if using) and cook for another 5 mins.

STEP 4 Add the tomatoes, spices and bay leaf, and season well. Bring to the boil and simmer for 15-20 mins, stirring often. Remove the bay leaf once it's done.

STEP 5 While the meat sauce is cooking, make up the white sauce. Warm the olive oil in a clean saucepan over a medium heat. Add the flour, whisking constantly to make a smooth paste.

STEP 6 Gradually add the milk while whisking to stop any lumps forming. Keep stirring until the sauce thickens – this can take around 5-10 mins. Once thickened, stir in the egg yolks, salt, pepper, nutmeg and cheese. Keep whisking to ensure the eggs don't scramble.

STEP 7 To assemble: drizzle some olive oil on the bottom of a large rectangular baking dish. Cover the base with the sliced potatoes, then add a layer of aubergines and courgettes – using about half of them. Pour over the meat ragu and spread it evenly. Layer the remaining aubergines and courgettes on top, then cover with the white sauce. Sprinkle over the grated cheese and herbs (if using), and arrange the sliced tomatoes across the top.

STEP 8 Bake in the middle shelf of the oven for about 45 mins to 1 hr, or until the cheese turns golden-brown. Allow the moussaka to cool for at least 20 mins before serving so the dish can set slightly.

INGREDIENTS

OLIVE OIL, FOR FRYING
SEA SALT AND FRESHLY GROUND PEPPER

FOR THE FIRST LAYER:
3 AUBERGINES/EGGPLANTS, CUT INTO ROUNDS
2 COURGETTES/ZUCCHINIS, CUT INTO ROUNDS
3 FLOURY, SMALL POTATOES, PEELED AND SLICED INTO THIN ROUNDS

FOR THE MEAT SAUCE:
1 RED ONION, CHOPPED
2 GARLIC CLOVES, MINCED
1TSP THYME
1TSP SUGAR
500G | 17.6OZ LAMB MINCE
2TBSP TOMATO PURÉE/PASTE
1 GLASS RED WINE (OPTIONAL)
400G | 14OZ TIN CHOPPED TOMATOES
1/2 TSP NUTMEG
1TSP GROUND CINNAMON
1 BAY LEAF

FOR THE WHITE SAUCE:
120ML | 4FLOZ OLIVE OIL
85G | 3OZ PLAIN FLOUR
900ML | 30.4FLOZ MILK
2 EGG YOLKS
1/2 TSP NUTMEG
150G | 5.3OZ KEFALOTYRI OR GRAVIERA CHEESE (OR PARMESAN IF NOT AVAILABLE)

FOR THE TOPPING:
1 HANDFUL GRATED KEFALOTYRI OR GRAVIERA CHEESE
1/2-1TSP DRIED MIXED HERBS (OPTIONAL)
1 LARGE TOMATO, SLICED INTO ROUNDS

MAIN MEALS

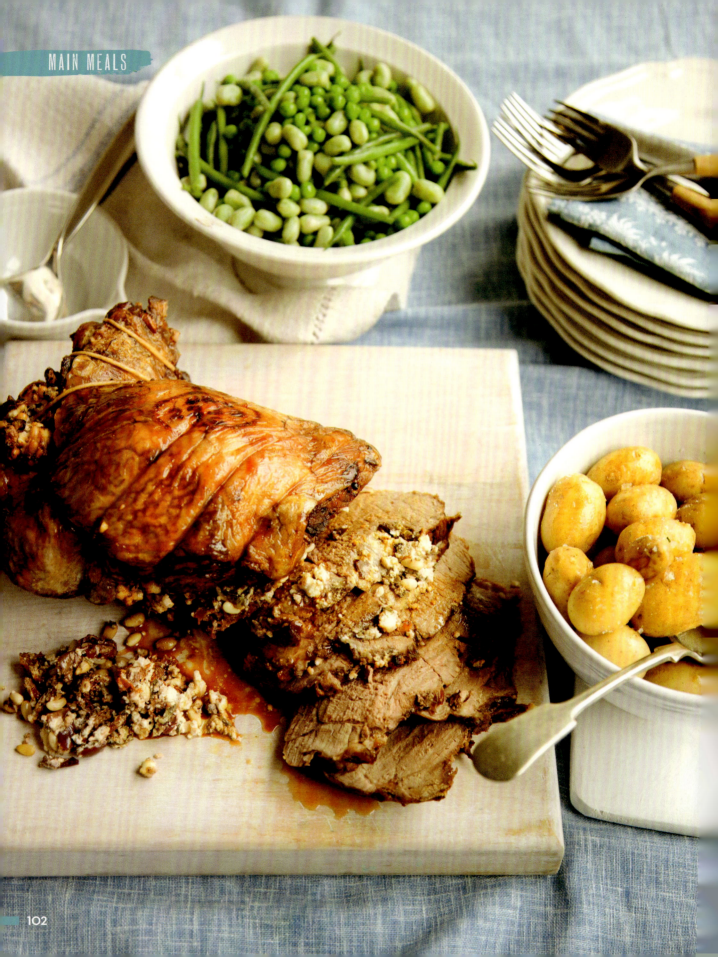

SERVINGS 8 **PREP TIME 20–25 MINS** **COOK TIME 1 HR 40 MINS**

MEDITERRANEAN LAMB WITH FETA STUFFING

THE FETA CONTRASTS PERFECTLY WITH THE RICHNESS OF THE LAMB AND GIVES IT A PLEASANT SALTINESS

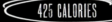

425 CALORIES

INGREDIENTS

- 200G | 7OZ FETA CHEESE
- 4-5 SPRIGS OREGANO, LEAVES ONLY, ROUGHLY CHOPPED
- 50G | 1.8OZ PITTED BLACK OLIVES IN OIL, DRAINED AND CHOPPED
- 50G | 1.8OZ SUN-DRIED TOMATOES, CHOPPED
- 35G | 1.2OZ PINE NUTS
- FRESHLY GROUND PEPPER
- 1 LEG OF LAMB, AROUND 1.8-2KG | 4-4.4LB, BUTTERFLIED

YOU WILL NEED:
BUTCHER'S STRING
A LARGE ROASTING TIN, LINED WITH FOIL

STEP 1 Preheat the oven to 180°C (160°C fan) | 350°F | gas 4. Roughly chop the feta, then put in a bowl with the oregano, olives, tomatoes and pine nuts. Season with pepper (but no salt – the feta will be salty enough). Mix it all together well, then open out the lamb, skin side down, and stuff the mixture into the cuts and opening. Use your hands and push it in really well.

STEP 2 String up the lamb. You may find it easier to cut several pieces of butcher's string at intervals and just knot them to secure the stuffing. Weigh the lamb to calculate the cooking time. Put in the roasting tin and roast for 40 mins per kg (or 18 mins per lb), plus an extra 20 mins. This will give you just-pink lamb.

TIP
You can buy ready boned-out lamb legs but they are often quite small, so it's worth ordering one from your butcher to have one of this size to serve 8.

Serve with new potatoes drizzled with olive oil, plus green beans, broad/fava beans and peas. Steam the potatoes and green veg until tender. This dish doesn't need any gravy, but a drizzle of pomegranate molasses would work well.

MAIN MEALS

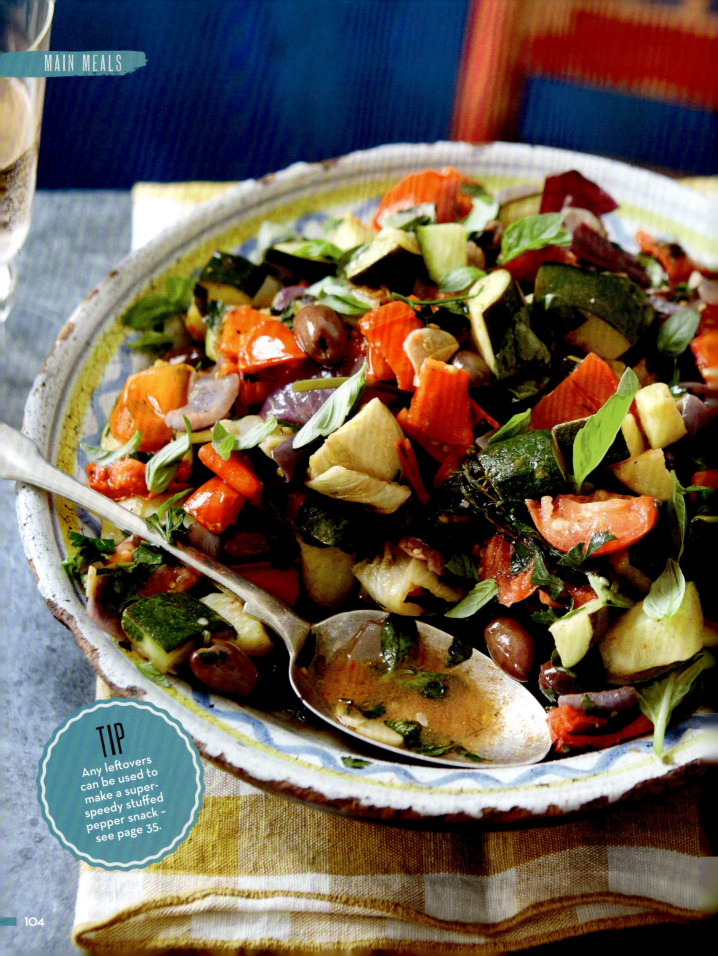

TIP
Any leftovers can be used to make a super-speedy stuffed pepper snack – see page 35.

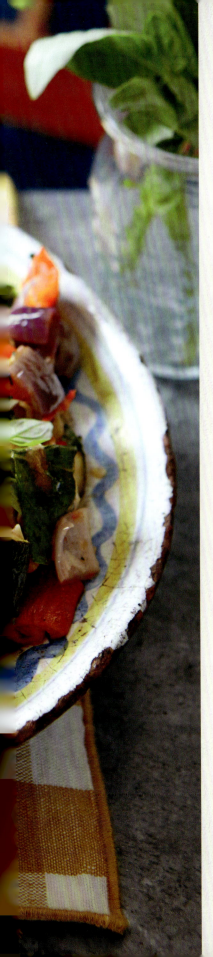

SERVINGS 4   PREP TIME 20-25 MINS   COOK TIME 30 MINS

SUMMER RATATOUILLE

FRESH TOMATOES AND GENEROUS QUANTITIES OF FRAGRANT HERBS MAKE THIS RATATOUILLE VIBRANT AND SUMMERY

200 CALORIES

INGREDIENTS

- 1 SMALL HEAD OF CELERY, ROUGHLY CHOPPED
- 3 RED BELL PEPPERS, ROUGHLY CHOPPED
- 2 ONIONS, ROUGHLY CHOPPED
- 1 SMALL FENNEL BULB, ROUGHLY CHOPPED
- 3TBSP OLIVE OIL
- 2 COURGETTES/ZUCCHINIS, ROUGHLY CHOPPED
- A FEW SPRIGS FRESH THYME
- 3 GARLIC CLOVES, THINLY SLICED
- ½ TBSP CASTER SUGAR
- 130G | 4.5OZ PITTED BLACK OLIVES
- 270G | 9.5OZ CHERRY TOMATOES, QUARTERED
- 1 HANDFUL EACH OF BASIL AND FLAT-LEAF/ITALIAN PARSLEY, LEAVES ONLY

STEP 1 Preheat the oven to 180°C (160°C fan) | 350°F | gas 4. Toss the celery, red peppers, onions and fennel in 2tbsp olive oil on a baking tray. Roast for 10 mins, until just soft. Add the courgettes and thyme, tossing to coat in the olive oil, and roast for another 10 mins. Remove from the oven and set aside.

STEP 2 Heat the remaining 1tbsp olive oil in a large frying pan over a medium heat. Fry the garlic until just golden. Add the roasted vegetables, sugar, olives and cherry tomatoes. Cook over a medium heat for a further few mins, until the tomatoes are warmed through but still holding their shape. Remove from the heat, scatter with the basil and parsley, and serve.

© Getty Images

MAIN MEALS

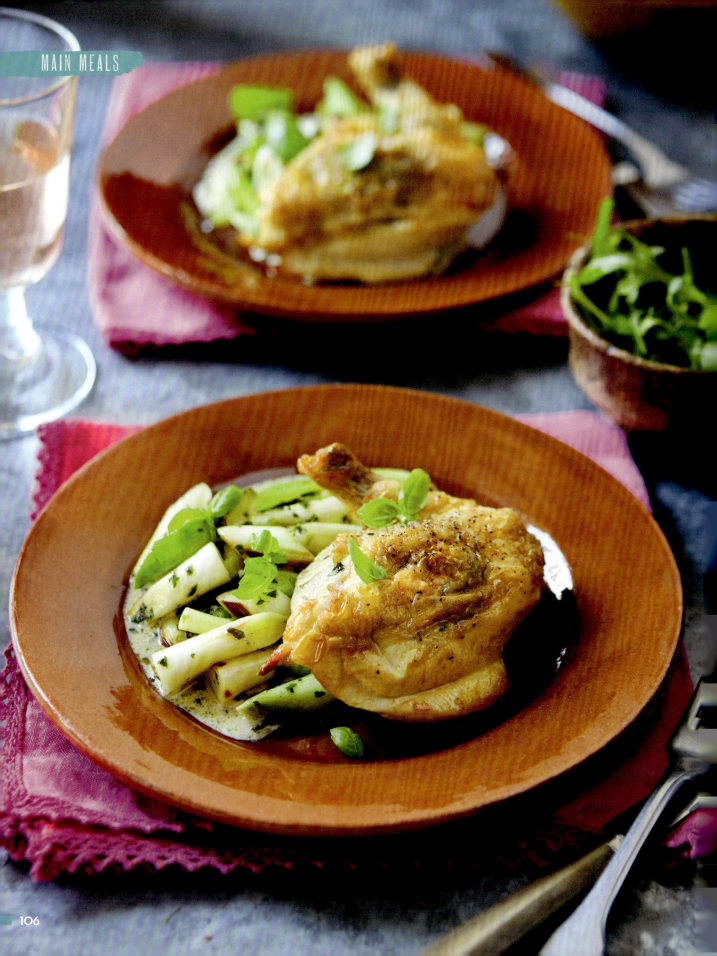

SERVINGS 4   PREP TIME 20-25 MINS   COOK TIME 20 MINS

CHICKEN STUFFED WITH BASIL

THIS IS AN EASY DISH AND A GREAT WAY TO JAZZ UP CHICKEN, PERFECT IF YOU HAVE A BIG POT OF BASIL IN THE GARDEN

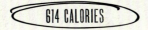

614 CALORIES

INGREDIENTS

4 CHICKEN SUPREMES
3TBSP OLIVE OIL
350G | 12.3OZ BABY LEEKS, TRIMMED AND SLICED
4TBSP CRÈME FRAÎCHE
SEA SALT AND FRESHLY GROUND PEPPER

FOR THE BASIL PURÉE:
3 GARLIC CLOVES, BASHED
2 HANDFULS OF FRESH BASIL
150ML | 5FLOZ EXTRA VIRGIN OLIVE OIL

YOU WILL NEED:
COCKTAIL STICKS

STEP 1 First, make the basil purée. Use a blender to whizz the ingredients together (including the basil stalks) with a good pinch of sea salt.

STEP 2 Preheat the oven to 200°C (180°C fan) | 400°F | gas 6. Carefully pull back the chicken skin without removing it. Make an incision in the centre thick part and spoon in some purée. Put back the skin and secure the end with a cocktail stick. Do this for all 4 pieces (you can do this ahead and leave them in the fridge overnight).

STEP 3 Put the chicken on an oiled baking tray, rub the skin with a little of the oil and sprinkle with sea salt and black pepper. Roast in the oven for about 20 mins or until cooked through.

STEP 4 While the chicken cooks, prepare the leeks. Heat the oil in a sauté pan and cook them for about 10-15 mins or until just softened. Add the crème fraîche and 3tbsp of the basil purée. Serve with the chicken with potatoes or crusty bread.

TIP

The basil purée will keep for a week in the fridge, and it's delicious added to a soup or to pasta.

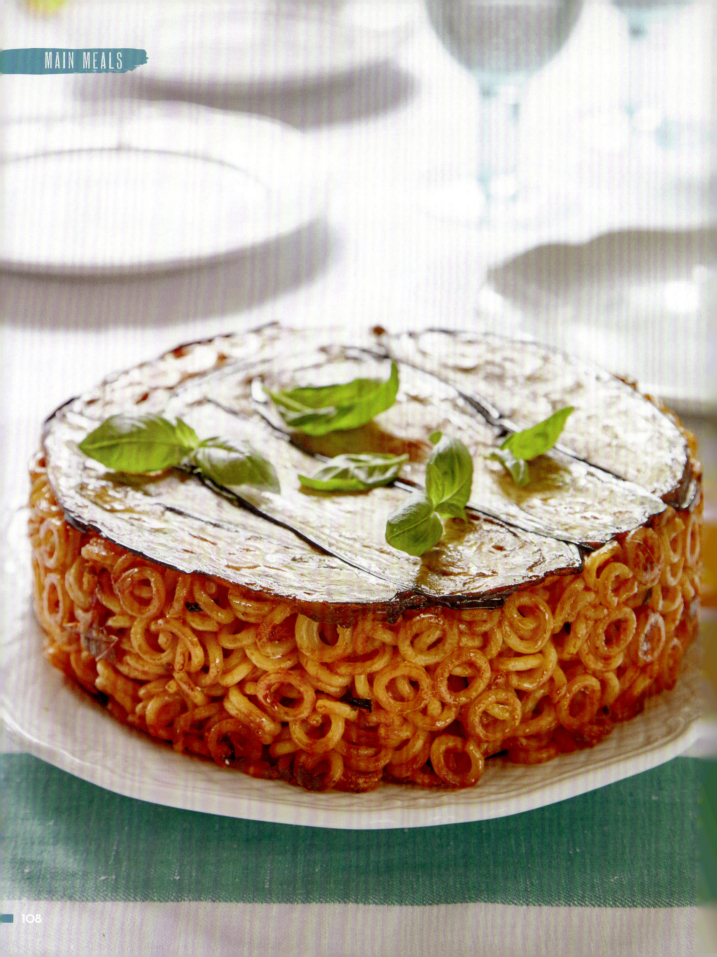

SERVINGS 8   PREP TIME 15-20 MINS   REST TIME 10 MINS   COOK TIME 1 HR 25 MINS

TIMBALLO SICILIANO

THIS SHOWSTOPPER TAKES ITS NAME FROM THE OLD FRENCH WORD FOR KETTLEDRUM – IT'S ESSENTIALLY A PIE MADE OF PASTA

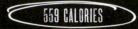
559 CALORIES

INGREDIENTS

FOR THE TOMATO SAUCE:
2TBSP OLIVE OIL
2 GARLIC CLOVES, CRUSHED
SMALL BUNCH BASIL
4X 400G | 14OZ TINS CHOPPED TOMATOES
1TSP CASTER SUGAR
SEA SALT AND FRESHLY GROUND PEPPER

FOR THE PASTA:
500G | 17.6OZ ANELLINI HOOP PASTA, MACARONI OR RIGATONI
6TBSP OLIVE OIL
100G | 3.5OZ PARMESAN, FINELY GRATED

FOR THE FILLING:
OLIVE OIL, FOR FRYING
4 AUBERGINES/EGGPLANTS, 1 SLICED LENGTHWAYS, 3 CHOPPED INTO CUBES
100G | 3.5OZ PARMESAN, FINELY GRATED

YOU WILL NEED:
20CM | 8" ROUND CAKE TIN, LIGHTLY GREASED WITH OLIVE OIL

STEP 1 Make the tomato sauce by heating the oil in a pan with the garlic for a few mins. Add most of the basil and cook for 30 secs, then add the tomatoes and sugar. Season and simmer for 25 mins, or until reduced by half. Remove from heat.

STEP 2 Bring a separate pan of water to the boil and cook the pasta for 10-12 mins, until al dente. Drain, return to the pan, add the olive oil and Parmesan, and stir in half of the tomato sauce.

STEP 3 For the filling, in a frying pan, heat 2cm | 0.75" oil and fry the aubergine slices (for the top of your timballo) and the cubed aubergine until golden. Add the cubed aubergine to the remaining tomato sauce and cook for 15 mins until reduced. Stir in the cheese.

STEP 4 Preheat the oven to 180°C (160°C fan) | 350°F | gas 4. To assemble, line the base of the tin with the aubergine slices. Add three-quarters of the pasta, making sure it lines the base and sides, leaving a gap in the centre to scoop in the aubergine and tomato sauce mix, then place the remaining pasta on top.

STEP 5 Bake for 20-25 mins, leave to stand for 10 mins, then turn out onto a platter. Top with a few basil leaves before serving.

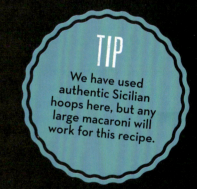
TIP
We have used authentic Sicilian hoops here, but any large macaroni will work for this recipe.

MAIN MEALS

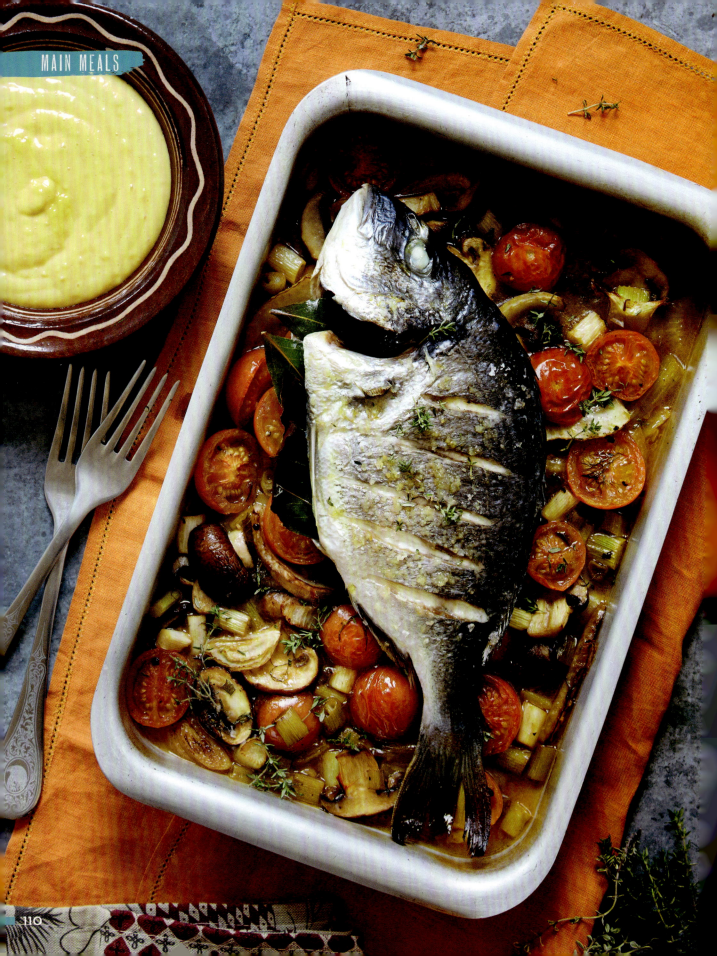

SERVINGS 2　　**PREP TIME** 15-20 MINS　　**COOK TIME** 35 MINS

FISHERMAN'S SEA BREAM WITH AIOLI

YOU CAN ALSO USE SEA BASS FOR THIS EASY RECIPE

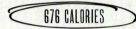

676 CALORIES

INGREDIENTS

2 TBSP OLIVE OIL
1 SMALL BULB FENNEL, CHOPPED
150G | 5.3OZ BROWN CAP MUSHROOMS, THICKLY SLICED
200G | 7OZ SMALL TOMATOES, HALVED
PINCH OF SAFFRON THREADS
150ML | 5FLOZ DRY WHITE WINE
1 SEA BREAM, APPROXIMATELY 750-800G | 26.5-28.2OZ, SCALED AND GUTTED
5 FRESH BAY LEAVES
A FEW SPRIGS OF FRESH THYME
SEA SALT AND FRESHLY GROUND PEPPER

FOR THE AIOLI:
3 GARLIC CLOVES, CRUSHED
1 LEMON, JUICE ONLY
2 EGG YOLKS
250ML | 8.5FLOZ OLIVE OIL

STEP 1 Start by making the aioli. Mix together the garlic, lemon and egg yolks with a good pinch of salt. Gradually whisk in the oil and keep whisking (an electric hand whisk is best) until thickened. Check for seasoning – it should be garlicky, but you may want to add more salt or lemon. Set aside, covered in the fridge.

STEP 2 Preheat the oven to 220°C (200°C fan) | 425°F | gas 7. Gently warm the olive oil in a sauté pan and cook the fennel for 10 mins until slightly softened. Add the mushrooms and cook for a few mins. Put into a shallow roasting tin, and add the tomatoes, saffron and white wine. Season well. Stuff the cavity of the bream with the bay leaves.

STEP 3 Put the bream on top of the tomato mixture then bake in the oven for about 15 mins or until the fish is cooked through. Serve the aioli on the side. This is delicious served with new potatoes.

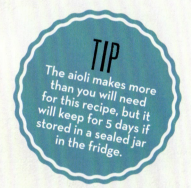

TIP
The aioli makes more than you will need for this recipe, but it will keep for 5 days if stored in a sealed jar in the fridge.

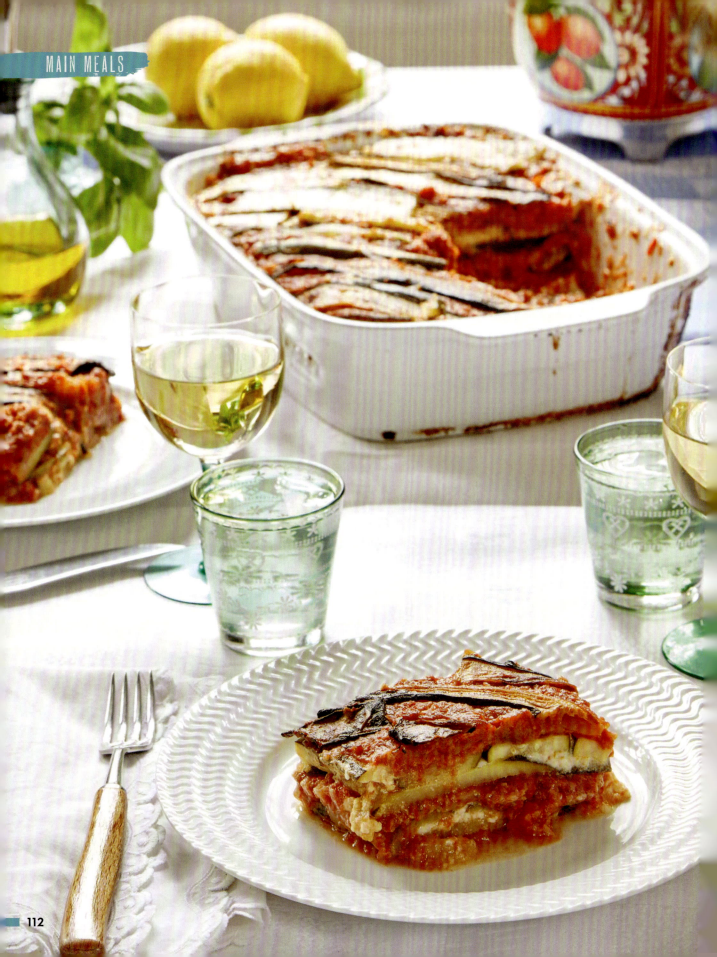

SERVINGS 4   PREP TIME 20 MINS   COOK TIME 1 HR 20 MINS

VEGETARIAN LASAGNE

A FABULOUS ALTERNATIVE TO THE MEAT VERSION, THIS RICH DISH WILL TAKE YOU STRAIGHT TO THE MEDITERRANEAN

826 CALORIES

INGREDIENTS

FOR THE TOMATO SAUCE:
4TBSP OLIVE OIL, PLUS EXTRA FOR FRYING
2 SMALL RED ONIONS, DICED
4 GARLIC CLOVES, SLICED
1KG | 2.2LB PASSATA/ TOMATO PURÉE
2TBSP TOMATO PURÉE/PASTE
2TBSP SHERRY VINEGAR
2TSP CASTER SUGAR
1 VEGETABLE STOCK CUBE

FOR THE FILLING:
4 COURGETTES/ZUCCHINIS, CUT INTO 0.5CM | 0.2" THICK STRIPS
1 AUBERGINE/EGGPLANT, CUT INTO 0.5CM | 0.2" THICK STRIPS
400G | 14OZ BALL MOZZARELLA

FOR THE WHITE SAUCE:
4TBSP OLIVE OIL
45G | 1.5OZ PLAIN FLOUR
1TSP NUTMEG
500ML | 17FLOZ MILK

FOR THE TOPPING:
40G | 1.4OZ PARMESAN, GRATED

STEP 1 For the tomato sauce, heat the olive oil in a pan, add the onions and cook for 5 mins over a medium heat. Add the garlic for a further 2 mins. Mix in the rest of the ingredients, bring to the boil, then turn down the heat to a gentle simmer for 40 mins, allowing the sauce to reduce.

STEP 2 While the tomato sauce cooks, preheat the oven to 180°C (160°C fan) | 350°F | gas 4. For the filling, brush a tiny amount of olive oil over a griddle pan and, in batches, cook the sliced vegetables for about 2 mins on each side until they are marked with chargrill stripes across them.

STEP 3 For the white sauce, warm the olive oil in a pan then add the flour and nutmeg, and whisk to a smooth paste. Add a little of the milk whisking until smooth. Whisk in the remaining milk and bring to the boil, whisking continuously, until you have a thick sauce.

STEP 4 Layer a third of the tomato sauce into an ovenproof dish, followed by a layer of vegetables, half of the mozzarella then half of the white sauce. Repeat and layer the remaining tomato sauce and vegetables.

STEP 5 Bake for 30 mins then add one last layer of aubergine, sprinkle on the Parmesan and cook for 10 mins more.

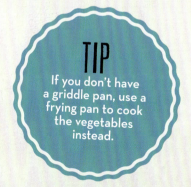

TIP
If you don't have a griddle pan, use a frying pan to cook the vegetables instead.

The tomato sauce can be bulked up with a drained jar of tuna.

MAIN MEALS

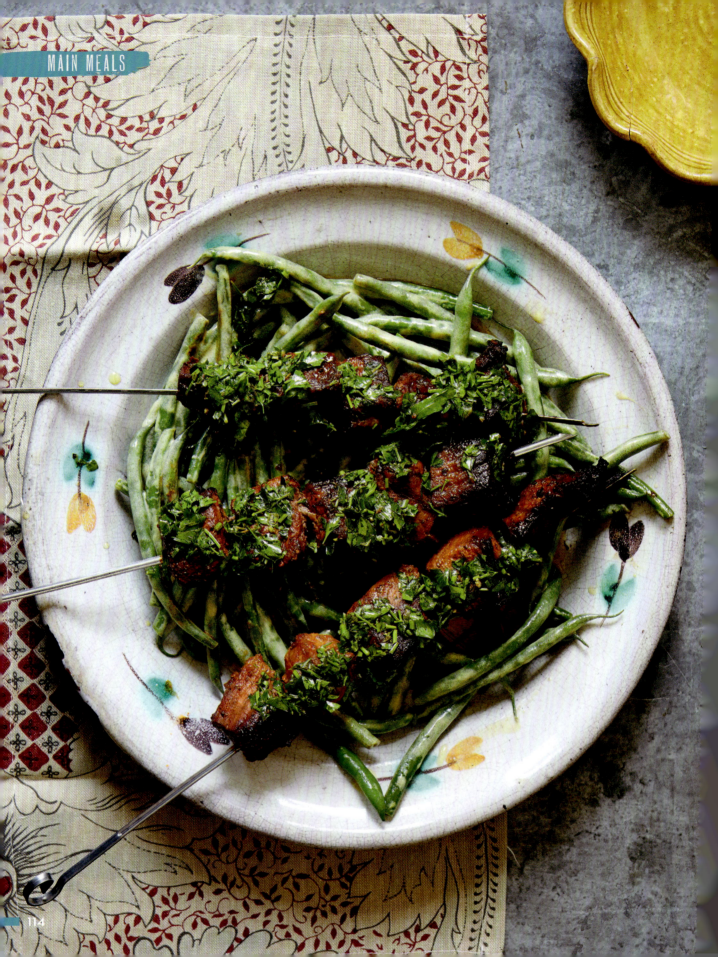

SERVINGS 6   PREP TIME 10 MINS   MARINATING TIME 3 HRS - OVERNIGHT   COOK TIME 20 MINS

PORTUGUESE-STYLE BEEF SKEWERS WITH FRENCH BEANS

THE HERBY 'SAUCE' IN THIS RECIPE WORKS WELL WITH ANY GRILL

506 CALORIES

INGREDIENTS

1.2KG | 2.6LB PIECE RUMP OR TOP RUMP
CRUSTY BREAD, TO SERVE

FOR THE MARINADE:
2TBSP SMOKED PAPRIKA
1TSP CAYENNE PEPPER
1TBSP CUMIN
1TBSP DRIED OREGANO
2TBSP OLIVE OIL
3TBSP RED WINE VINEGAR
3TBSP BROWN SUGAR

FOR THE SAUCE:
6TBSP FLAT-LEAF/ITALIAN PARSLEY, ROUGHLY CHOPPED
2TBSP FRESH OREGANO, LEAVES ONLY
4TBSP EXTRA VIRGIN OLIVE OIL
1 LEMON, JUICE ONLY

FOR THE BEANS:
300G | 10.5OZ FRENCH BEANS, TRIMMED
1TBSP DIJON MUSTARD
2TBSP RED WINE VINEGAR
100ML | 3.4FLOZ EXTRA VIRGIN OLIVE OIL

YOU WILL NEED:
METAL SKEWERS

STEP 1 Cut the beef into large chunks, trimming off any sinew. Mix together the marinade ingredients and add the beef, coating the meat thoroughly. Put into a bowl and leave to marinate in the fridge for at least 3 hrs or overnight.

STEP 2 Once marinated, thread the meat onto metal skewers. To make the sauce, simply whizz the ingredients together in a food processor. Cover and set aside.

STEP 3 Cook the beans until just tender, about 8 mins, then drain. Whisk the mustard and vinegar together then gradually whisk in the oil. Toss the vinaigrette into the warm beans.

STEP 4 Grill the skewers under the grill or on the barbecue for a few mins each side, until cooked to your liking. Spoon over the herb sauce and serve with the beans and plenty of crusty bread.

TIP
These skewers would be just as tasty with lamb or pork, but if limiting your red meat intake they would also be great with chicken, tuna or tofu.

MAIN MEALS

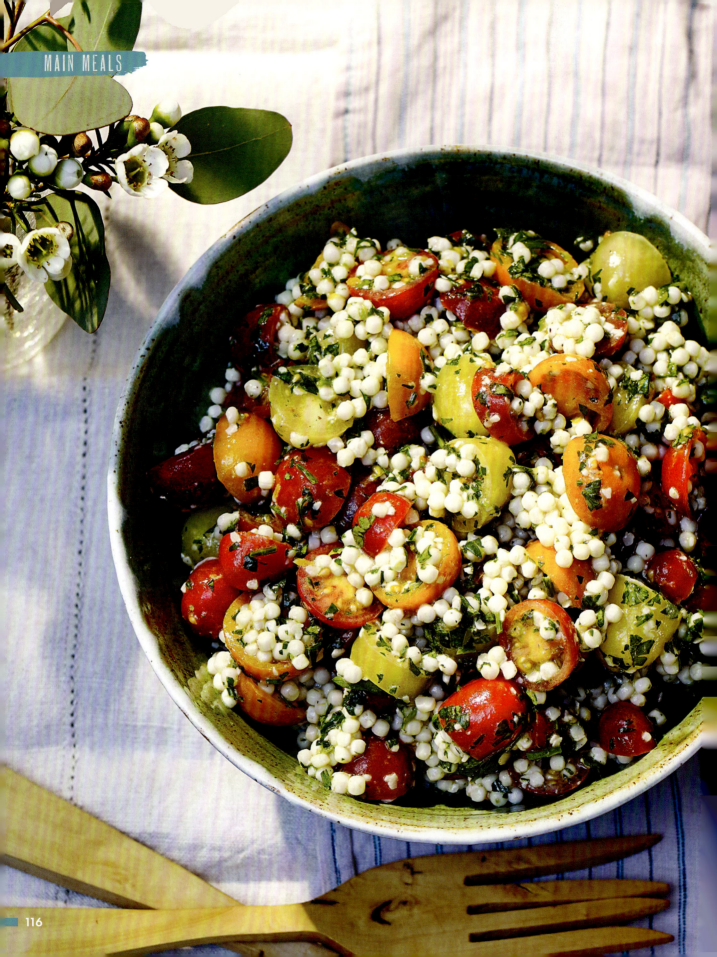

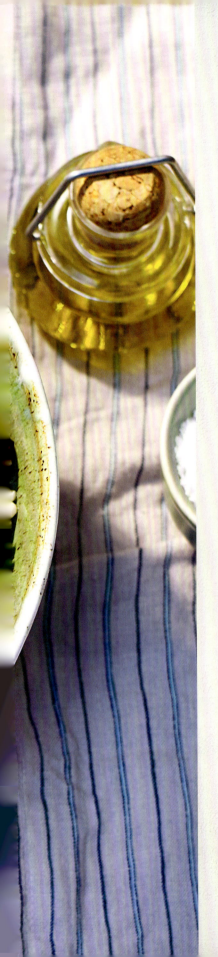

SERVINGS 6-8 | PREP TIME 10-15 MINS | REST TIME 10 MINS

TOMATO AND COUSCOUS SALAD

THIS DELICIOUS SALAD CONTAINS FEW INGREDIENTS BUT IT'S ALL ABOUT THE RIPENESS OF THE TOMATOES AND THE QUALITY OF THE OLIVE OIL

311-233 CALORIES

INGREDIENTS

- **250G | 8.8OZ** TOASTED COUSCOUS OR GIANT (ISRAELI) COUSCOUS
- **2** LEMONS, ZESTED AND JUICED
- **8TBSP** EXTRA VIRGIN OLIVE OIL
- **500G | 17.6OZ** CHERRY TOMATOES, HALVED
- **1** LARGE BUNCH FLAT-LEAF/ITALIAN PARSLEY, FINELY CHOPPED
- SEA SALT AND FRESHLY GROUND PEPPER

STEP 1 Put the couscous in a large bowl. Pour over boiling water to come about 2cm | 0.75" above the surface. Cover with cling film and leave to stand for 10 mins or until tender. Put into a colander and run under cold water. Put back into the bowl and add the lemon zest and juice, and the olive oil. Add plenty of seasoning.

STEP 2 Make sure your tomatoes are at room temperature (see tip). Stir them into the couscous with the chopped parsley and serve it immediately.

TIP
Raw tomatoes are best enjoyed at room temperature. When they are cold from the fridge, it deadens their flavour.

MAIN MEALS

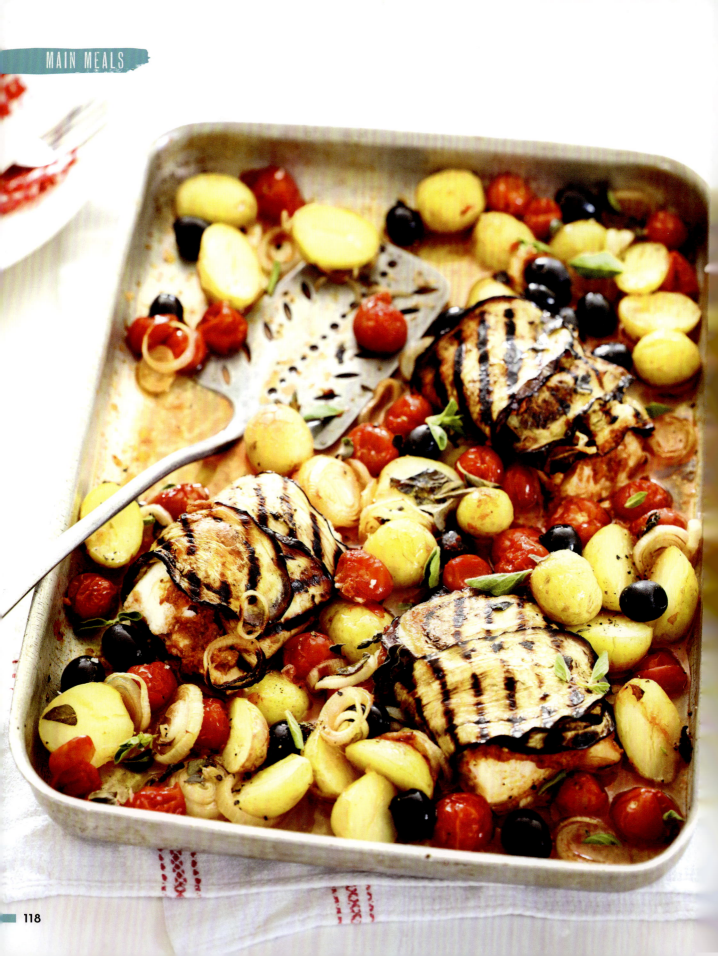

SERVINGS 4   PREP TIME 20 MINS   COOK TIME 30-35 MINS

PROVENÇAL FISH TRAYBAKE

MEDITERRANEAN FLAVOURS GO WELL WITH FISH – IT'S SUMMER ON A PLATE!

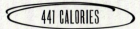

441 CALORIES

INGREDIENTS

- 600G | 1.3LB NEW POTATOES
- 1 LARGE AUBERGINE/EGGPLANT, SLICED 0.5CM | 0.2" THICK LENGTHWAYS
- 175ML | 5.9FLOZ WHITE WINE
- 3 SHALLOTS, SLICED
- 250G | 8.8OZ CHERRY TOMATOES, HALVED
- 80G | 2.8OZ PITTED BLACK OLIVES
- 2TBSP OLIVE OIL
- SEA SALT AND FRESHLY GROUND PEPPER
- A FEW SPRIGS OREGANO, FINELY CHOPPED
- 3TBSP SUNDRIED TOMATO PESTO
- 4X 150G | 5.3OZ THICK WHITE FISH FILLETS (SUCH AS COLEY), SKINNED AND BONED

STEP 1 Boil the potatoes until just tender, cool slightly and halve. Griddle or grill the aubergine for 2-3 mins each side until soft. Boil the wine for 2 mins until it has reduced by about a third.

STEP 2 Preheat the oven to 200°C (180°C fan) | 400°F | gas 6. Arrange the shallots, tomatoes, olives and potatoes in a large roasting tin and drizzle with the oil and wine. Season well with salt and pepper and scatter over half the oregano.

STEP 3 Spread the pesto onto one side of each fish fillet, scatter with the remaining oregano, then wrap each with a quarter of the aubergine slices and arrange in the roasting tin. Bake for 15-20 mins.

MAIN MEALS

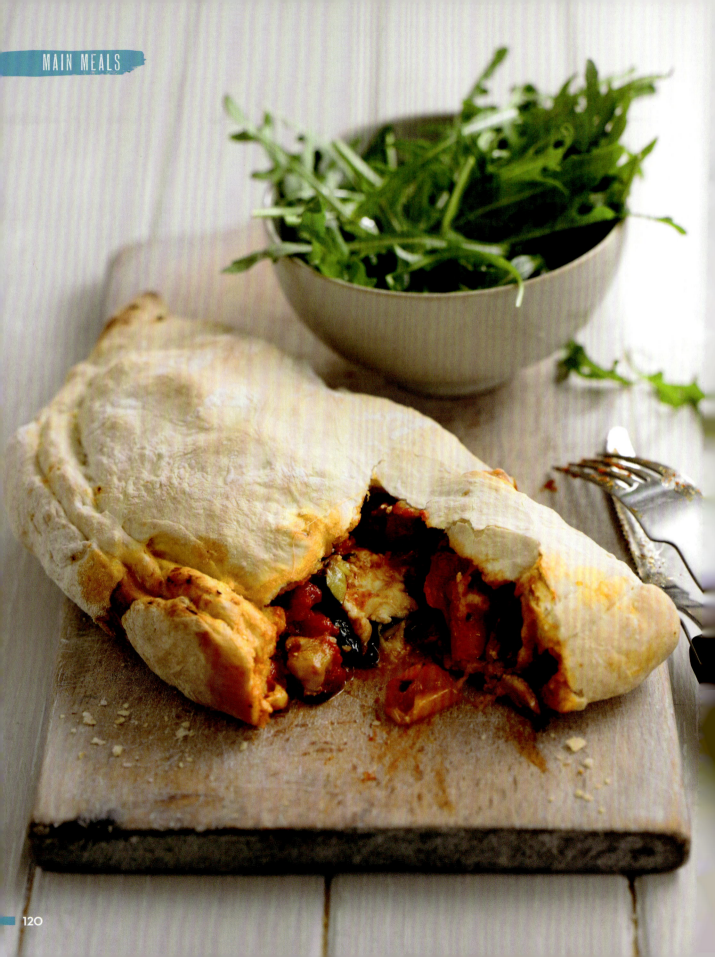

SERVINGS 2-4   **PREP TIME 15-20 MINS**   **COOK TIME 45-50 MINS**

MEDITERRANEAN VEGETABLE CALZONE

AN IRRESISTIBLE CROSS BETWEEN A PIZZA AND A CORNISH PASTY! THIS HEARTY DISH MAKES THE PERFECT COMFORT FOOD

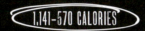
1,141-570 CALORIES

INGREDIENTS

750G | 26.5OZ FROZEN MEDITERRANEAN VEGETABLES
2 GARLIC CLOVES, CRUSHED
3TBSP OLIVE OIL
2TBSP SUN-DRIED TOMATO PASTE
SEA SALT AND FRESHLY GROUND PEPPER
560G | 19.8OZ CHILLED PIZZA DOUGH, DIVIDED IN HALF AND ROLLED OUT INTO TWO ROUNDS
150G | 5.3OZ MOZZARELLA CHEESE, DRAINED AND TORN INTO PIECES (OPTIONAL)
ROCKET/ARUGULA LEAVES, TO SERVE

STEP 1 Preheat the oven to 200°C (180°C fan) | 400°F | gas 6. Tip the frozen vegetables into a large roasting tray, spreading them out evenly. Scatter with garlic, drizzle with 1tbsp of the olive oil and roast for 25-30 mins, or until tender.

STEP 2 Mix the tomato paste and remaining oil together, add to the cooked vegetables and toss to coat. Season with salt and freshly ground pepper. Cool slightly.

STEP 3 Increase the oven to 220°C (200°C fan) | 425°F | gas 7. Spread half the vegetables over one half of each dough round, and brush the edges with water.

STEP 4 Top with pieces of mozzarella (if using) then fold each dough round in half and twist the edges to seal. Place on a baking tray and bake for 20 mins, until the dough is crisp.

STEP 5 If you are serving 4, slice each calzone in half. Serve with a simple salad of rocket leaves drizzled with some extra virgin olive oil.

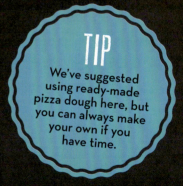

TIP
We've suggested using ready-made pizza dough here, but you can always make your own if you have time.

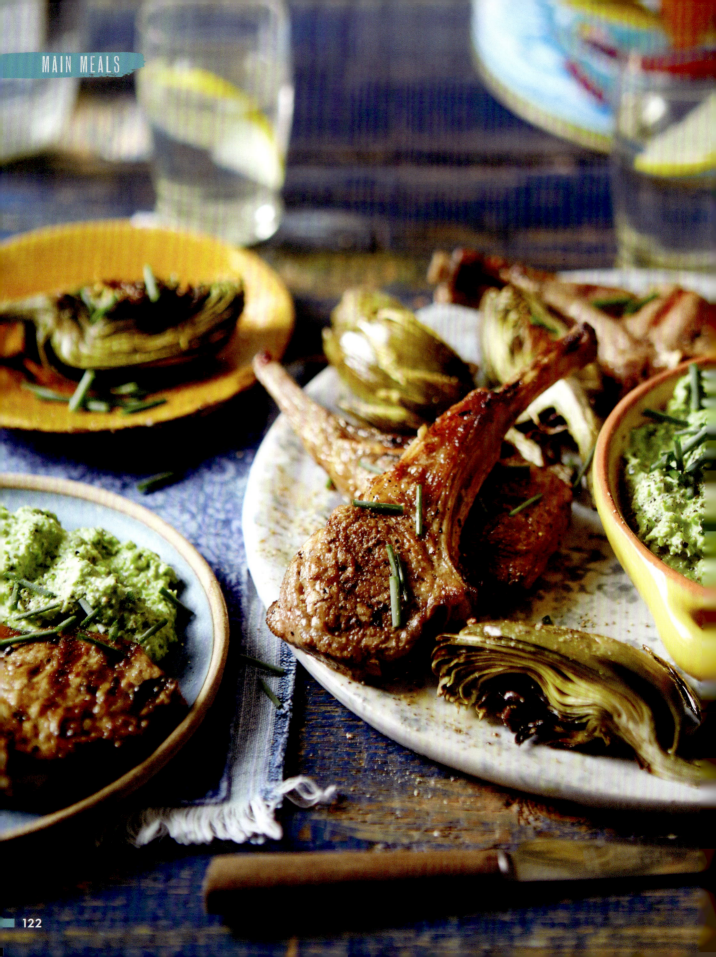
MAIN MEALS

SERVINGS 4   **PREP TIME 10 MINS**   **COOK TIME 30-35 MINS**

LAMB CUTLETS WITH PEA AND MINT PURÉE

CHOPS MAKE IDEAL FINGER FOOD, WITH EACH FINE BONE HOLDING A MOUTH-SIZED CHUNK OF SUCCULENT LAMB AT THE END

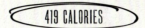

419 CALORIES

INGREDIENTS

- 2 GARLIC CLOVES, CRUSHED
- 1 LEMON, JUICE ONLY
- 2TBSP OLIVE OIL
- 8 LAMB CHOPS
- 2 SMALL GLOBE ARTICHOKES
- SEA SALT AND FRESHLY GROUND PEPPER

FOR THE PEA PURÉE:
- 250G | 8.8OZ FROZEN PEAS
- 15G | 0.5OZ FRESH MINT, LEAVES PICKED
- 5TBSP CRÈME FRAÎCHE
- 10G | 0.4OZ CHIVES (PLUS A FEW EXTRA, CHOPPED, TO SERVE)
- ½ LEMON, JUICE ONLY

STEP 1 Preheat the oven to 200°C (180°C fan) | 400°F | gas 6. In a non-metallic bowl, mix the garlic, lemon juice and half the oil, add the lamb chops and set aside to marinate while you prepare the rest.

STEP 2 Bring a pan of salted water to the boil and cook the artichokes for 10-15 mins until tender and a knife can be placed through them. Cut them into quarters, place on a baking tray and drizzle over the remaining oil. Cook for 10 mins in the oven until tender and crispy on the outside.

STEP 3 In a heatproof bowl, cover the peas with just-boiled water and leave to stand for 2 mins. Drain, then add to a food processor with the mint, crème fraîche, chives, lemon juice and seasoning. Whizz until smooth and adjust the seasoning to taste.

STEP 4 Heat a wide pan over a high heat and cook the lamb chops for 3 mins, fat side down, and then 3-4 mins each side, until browned – you may need to do this in batches. Warm the purée through and serve with the lamb and artichokes, scattered with the remaining chives.

TIP
You could use small pork chops for this recipe too. Perfect for al fresco entertaining – instead of cooking on a frying pan, just throw on the barbecue!

The lamb's delicate flavour pairs well with this seasonal pea sauce, which makes a wonderful dip too.

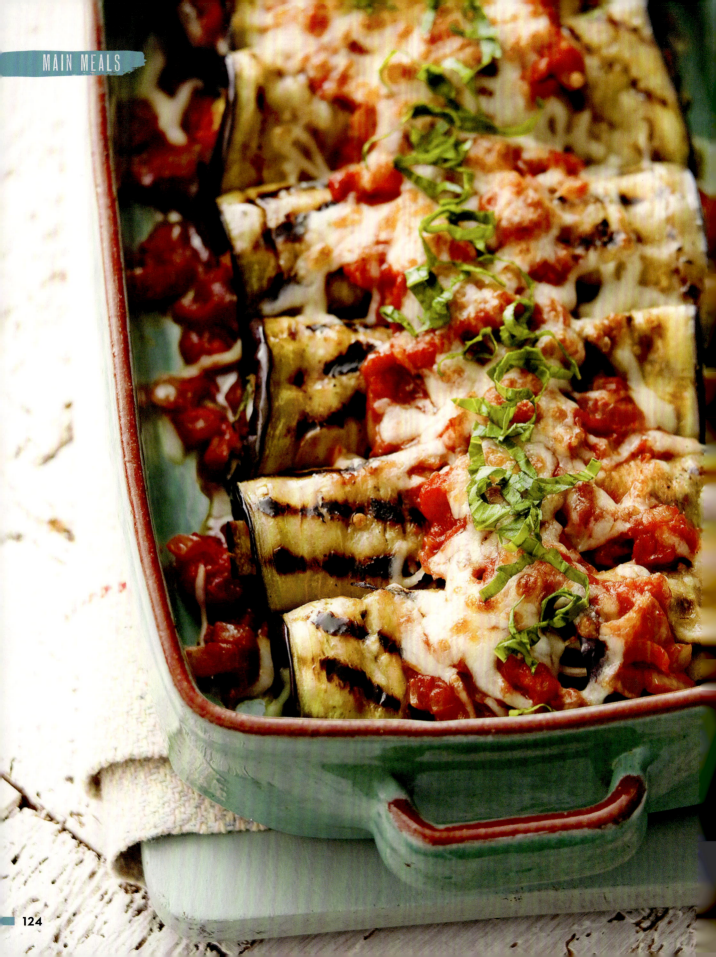
MAIN MEALS

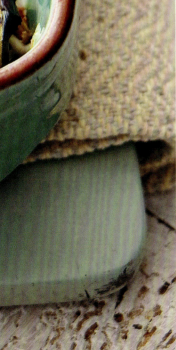

SERVINGS 4   PREP TIME 20-25 MINS   COOK TIME 20-25 MINS

MEDITERRANEAN VEG ROLLS

THIS DISH MAKES FOR A LOVELY MEAT-FREE SUPPER

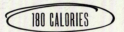

180 CALORIES

INGREDIENTS

- 3TBSP OLIVE OIL
- 1 ONION, CHOPPED
- 1-2 GARLIC CLOVES
- 400G | 14OZ TIN CHOPPED TOMATOES
- 1TSP DRIED OREGANO
- SEA SALT AND FRESHLY GROUND PEPPER
- 2 LARGE AUBERGINES/EGGPLANTS
- 60G | 2OZ MOZZARELLA, GRATED
- 10 BASIL LEAVES, SHREDDED

STEP 1 Heat 1tbsp of the oil and fry the onion for 3 mins. Add the garlic and cook for a further 5 mins. Stir in the chopped tomatoes and oregano and simmer, uncovered, for 10-15 mins, until thickened. Season with salt and ground black pepper.

STEP 2 Cut each aubergine lengthways into 8 thin slices. Pick out the largest 12 slices. Brush these on both sides with the oil, and griddle or grill in batches until browned. Set aside. Griddle or grill the rest of the aubergine slices, then chop them and put in a bowl.

STEP 3 Add 4tbsp of the tomato sauce mixture to the chopped aubergine, and mix well. Spoon half the remaining tomato sauce into the base of a baking dish.

STEP 4 Preheat the oven to 200°C (180°C fan) | 400°F | gas 6. Lay the aubergine slices out on a board and divide the filling between them. Sprinkle with half the grated mozzarella and half the shredded basil leaves. Roll each slice up.

STEP 5 Pack the rolls in the dish, seam-side down. Spoon the remaining sauce over the top and sprinkle with the remaining mozzarella. Bake in the oven for 20 mins. Sprinkle with the rest of the shredded basil to serve.

MAIN MEALS

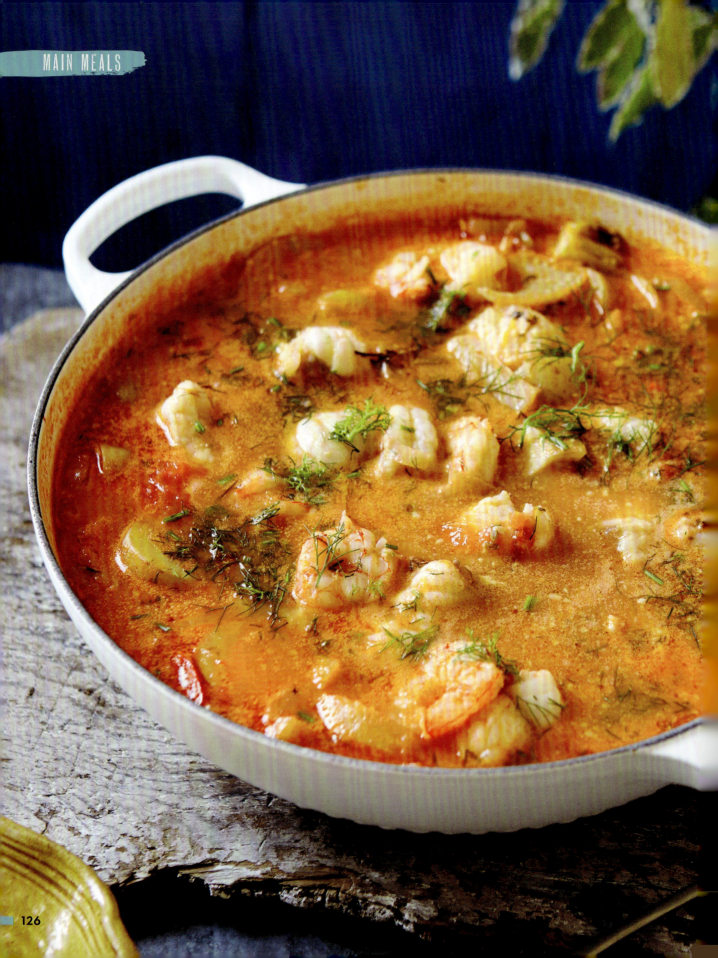

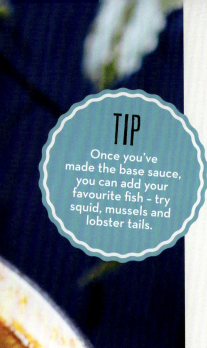

SERVINGS 6-8 | PREP TIME 10-15 MINS | COOK TIME 50 MINS - 1 HR

CATALAN FISH STEW

THIS ONE IS REALLY SIMPLE. YOU CAN MIX AND MATCH THE FISH AND IT'S ALL IN ONE POT – FABULOUS!

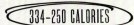
334-250 CALORIES

TIP
Once you've made the base sauce, you can add your favourite fish – try squid, mussels and lobster tails.

INGREDIENTS

- **2TBSP** OLIVE OIL
- **3** ONIONS, CHOPPED
- **1 LARGE BULB FENNEL**, CHOPPED (RESERVE THE FRONDS TO GARNISH)
- **2** GARLIC CLOVES, CRUSHED
- **1 PINCH** CHILLI FLAKES
- **400G | 14OZ** TIN CHOPPED TOMATOES
- **2TSP** FENNEL SEEDS
- **2** BAY LEAVES
- **750ML | 25.4FLOZ** FISH STOCK
- **250ML | 8.5FLOZ** WHITE WINE
- **500G | 17.6OZ** NEW POTATOES, UNPEELED AND THICKLY SLICED
- **1KG | 2.2LB** WHITE FISH, SUCH AS MONKFISH OR HAKE, CUT INTO CHUNKS
- **300G | 10.5OZ** LARGE PRAWNS
- SEA SALT AND FRESHLY GROUND PEPPER

STEP 1 Heat the olive oil a large pan then gently sweat the onions and fennel together for 20 mins. Add the garlic and cook for a few mins, then add the chilli, tomatoes, fennel seeds, bay, fish stock and white wine. Bring to the boil then add the potatoes and turn down to a simmer for about 20 mins or until the potatoes are tender.

STEP 2 Add the fish and prawns, season well and simmer for 5 mins or so until the fish is cooked. Scatter over the chopped fennel fronds and serve.

MAIN MEALS

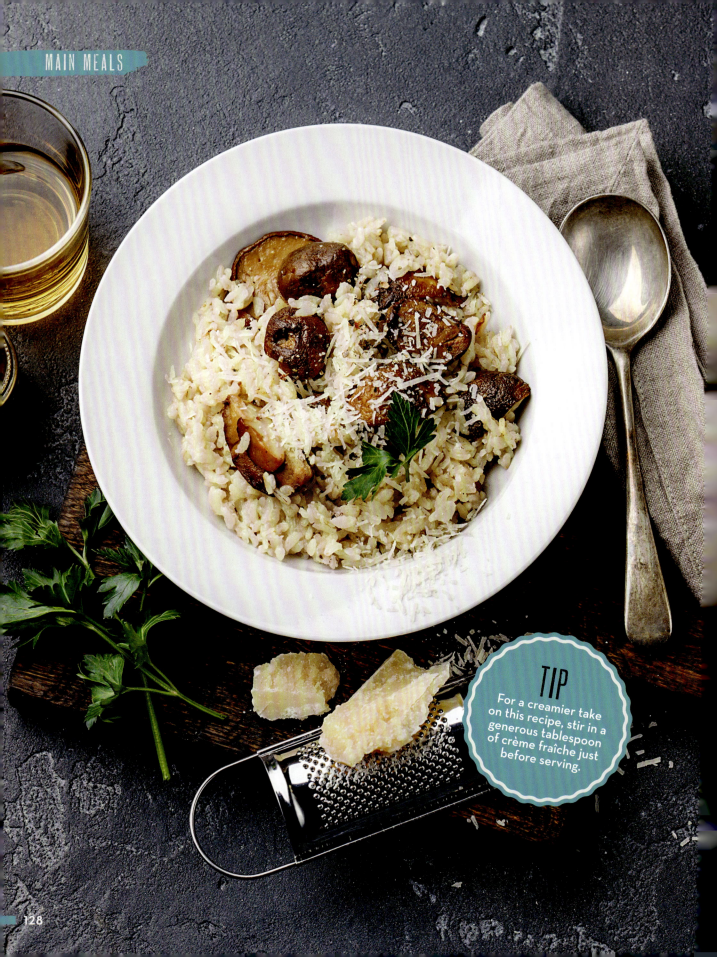

TIP
For a creamier take on this recipe, stir in a generous tablespoon of crème fraîche just before serving.

SERVINGS 4   PREP TIME 10 MINS   COOK TIME 30-35 MINS

RISOTTO AL FUNGHI

THIS HEARTY, FLAVOURSOME ITALIAN DISH IS SURPRISINGLY SIMPLE

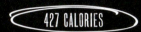
427 CALORIES

INGREDIENTS

- **2TBSP** OLIVE OIL
- **1** ONION, DICED
- **2** GARLIC CLOVES, DICED
- **250G | 8.8OZ** CHESTNUT MUSHROOMS, HALF DICED, HALF SLICED
- SEA SALT AND FRESHLY GROUND PEPPER
- **300G | 10.5OZ** ARBORIO RICE
- **200ML | 6.8FLOZ** WHITE WINE
- **1.2L | 2.5PT** CHICKEN STOCK
- **2TBSP** EXTRA VIRGIN OLIVE OIL
- **1TBSP** PARMESAN, GRATED, PLUS EXTRA TO SERVE
- FRESH PARSLEY, TO GARNISH

STEP 1 On a low heat, gently warm the olive oil in a large saucepan.

STEP 2 Add the onion to the saucepan and fry until it is soft and semi-translucent. Add the garlic and all the mushrooms, and fry for another 5 mins, then season to taste with salt and pepper.

STEP 3 Stir in all of the arborio rice to lightly toast. Fry for 1 min or so, but stir frequently to ensure the rice doesn't burn.

STEP 4 Turn the heat to medium, add in the wine and let it bubble away. The key to a good risotto is to keep stirring, ensuring that the rice is evenly cooked.

STEP 5 Once the wine has almost completely evaporated, add in a ladleful (around 100ml | 3.4 floz) of stock. *Do not* add in all of the stock at once, as this will ruin the texture.

STEP 6 When each ladleful of stock has been absorbed by the rice, add another. Keep stirring frequently to ensure that none of the rice sticks to the bottom of the pan.

STEP 7 As you reach the final quarter of your stock, keep checking the risotto's texture – it should be a sticky consistency. If you use up your stock and the risotto is still incomplete, add extra water in 2tbsp servings. When it's done, stir through the extra virgin olive oil and parmesan.

STEP 8 Add a sprig of fresh parsley and sprinkle with more parmesan to serve.

MAIN MEALS

TIP
This recipe also works with fresh tuna steaks instead of salmon. For thicker steaks you may have to bake for a few mins longer at step 1.

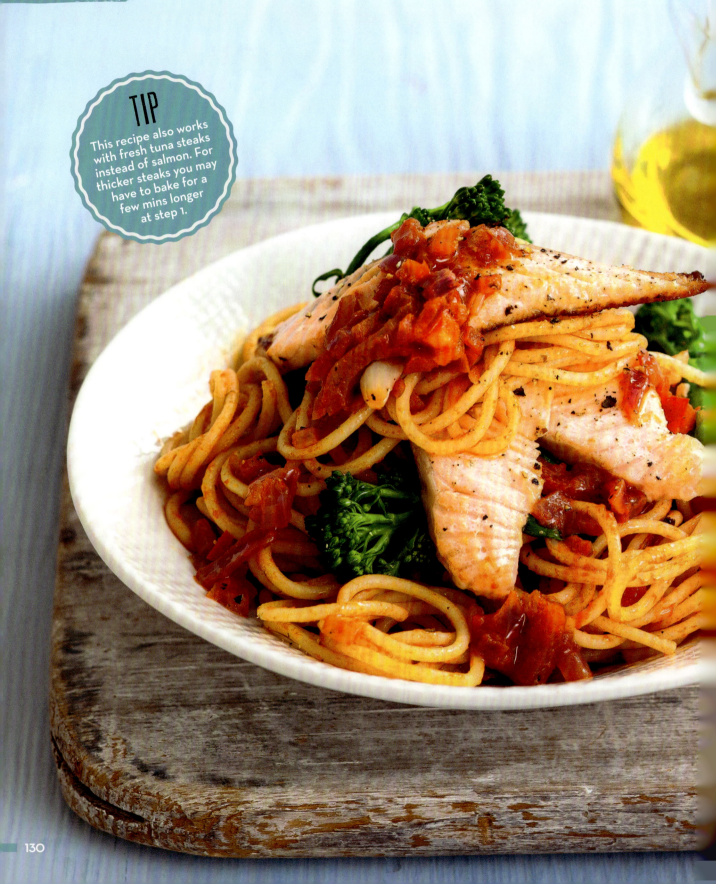

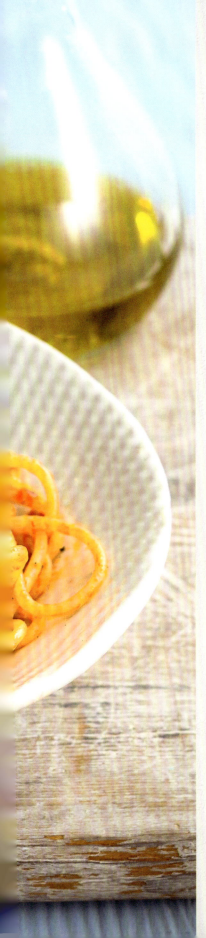

SERVINGS 4   **PREP TIME** 10 MINS   **COOK TIME** 30 MINS

SALMON & SPAGHETTI BOLOGNESE

PACKED FULL OF HEALTHY OMEGA-3, THIS DISH IS JUST AS TASTY AS IT IS HEALTHY

445 CALORIES

INGREDIENTS

- 250G | 8.8OZ SALMON FILLET, SLICED
- SEA SALT AND FRESHLY GROUND PEPPER
- 1 LEMON, ZESTED AND JUICED
- 2TBSP OLIVE OIL
- 1X 28G | 1OZ CONCENTRATED VEG STOCK
- 250G | 8.8OZ SPAGHETTI
- 150G | 5.3OZ TENDERSTEM BROCCOLI/BROCCOLINI
- 1 ONION, CHOPPED
- 2 GARLIC CLOVES, CRUSHED
- 1 RED BELL PEPPER, CHOPPED
- 200G | 7OZ PASSATA/TOMATO PURÉE

STEP 1 Preheat the oven to 200°C (180°C fan) | 400°F | gas 6. Put the salmon on a non-stick baking tray. Season generously with salt and freshly ground black pepper and sprinkle over lemon zest and juice, and 1tsp olive oil. Bake for 10 mins.

STEP 2 Meanwhile, add the concentrated vegetable stock to a pan of water, bring to the boil, add the spaghetti and cook for 10 mins. Add the broccoli for the final 3 mins of cooking time.

STEP 3 Heat the remaining oil in a frying pan, add the onion, garlic and pepper, and simmer gently for 5 mins. Add the passata and simmer for a few mins.

STEP 4 Drain the pasta and broccoli, and combine with the sauce. Serve topped with the salmon.

MAIN MEALS

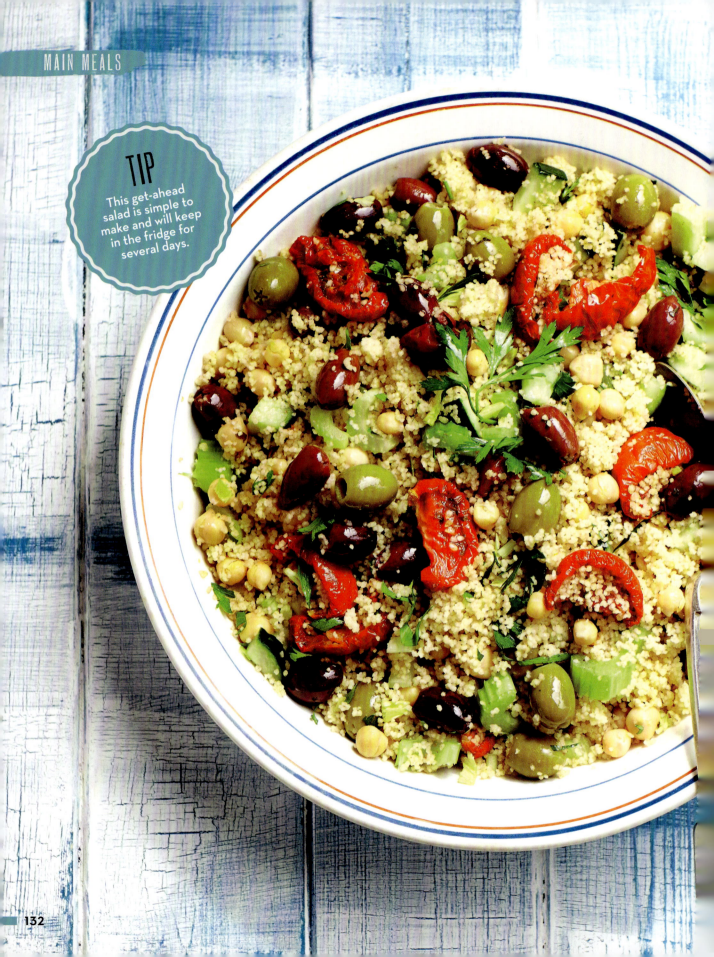

TIP
This get-ahead salad is simple to make and will keep in the fridge for several days.

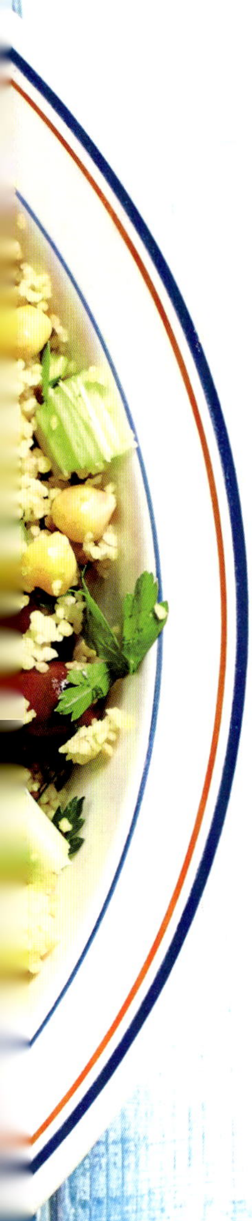

SERVINGS 6 **PREP TIME** 5 MINS **COOK TIME** 10 MINS

COUSCOUS AND CHICKPEA SALAD

SIMPLY SOAK THE COUSCOUS IN STOCK THEN MIX IN THE OTHER INGREDIENTS

338 CALORIES

INGREDIENTS

- 1X 28G | 1OZ CONCENTRATED VEGETABLE STOCK (SUCH AS KNORR STOCK POT)
- 150G | 5.3OZ COUSCOUS
- 400G | 14OZ TIN CHICKPEAS, DRAINED
- 225G | 8OZ PITTED MARINATED OLIVES, DRAINED
- 200G | 7OZ SUN-BLUSHED TOMATOES, DRAINED
- 3 STICKS OF CELERY, CHOPPED
- 2 TBSP CHOPPED PARSLEY
- SALT AND FRESHLY GROUND PEPPER

FOR THE FRENCH DRESSING:
- 1 TSP DIJON MUSTARD
- 2 TBSP WHITE WINE VINEGAR
- 6 TBSP EXTRA VIRGIN OLIVE OIL
- 1 PINCH SUGAR (OPTIONAL)

STEP 1 Put 150ml | 5floz boiling water into a pan and add the concentrated vegetable stock. Heat and stir to dissolve. Add the couscous and turn off the heat. Leave for 10 mins, to absorb the water. Tip the couscous into a large bowl and leave to cool.

STEP 2 Meanwhile, prepare the French dressing by whisking all the dressing ingredients together in a small bowl, season to taste and set aside.

STEP 3 Once the couscous has cooled, stir in the chickpeas, olives, sun-blushed tomatoes, celery, parsley and the French dressing, then season to taste. Stir everything together and either serve or chill until needed.

MAIN MEALS

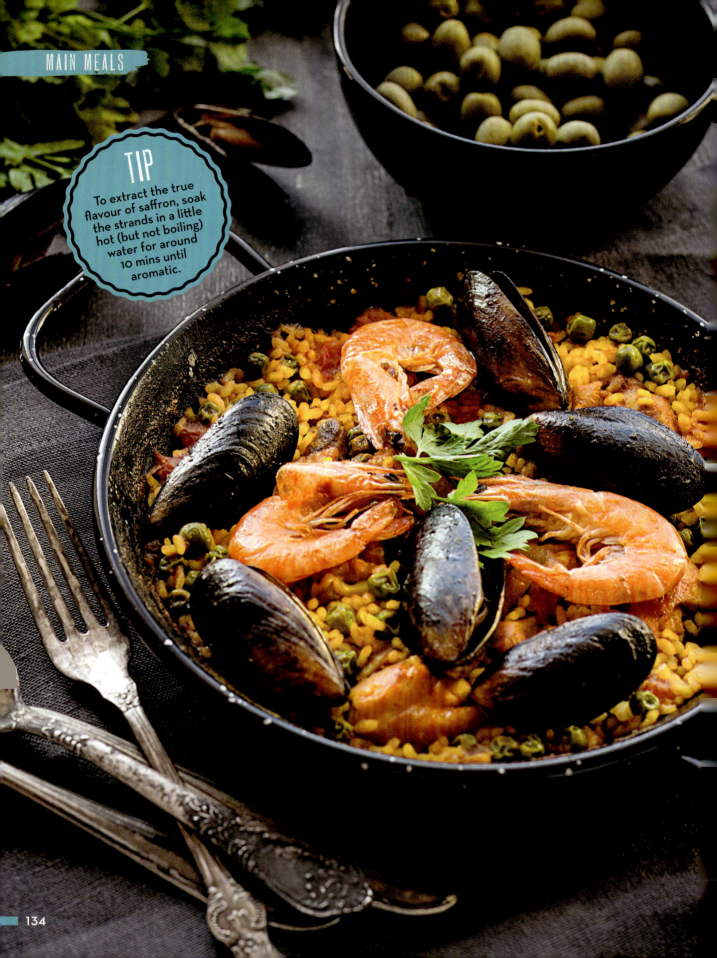

TIP
To extract the true flavour of saffron, soak the strands in a little hot (but not boiling) water for around 10 mins until aromatic.

SERVINGS 4 **PREP TIME 10 MINS** **COOK TIME 45 MINS**

PAELLA

THIS DELICIOUS BLEND OF CHICKEN, CHORIZO AND SEAFOOD IN AROMATIC RICE IS A MODERN TWIST ON A SPANISH CLASSIC

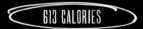

613 CALORIES

INGREDIENTS

- 2 TBSP OLIVE OIL
- 4 SKINLESS, BONELESS CHICKEN THIGHS
- SEA SALT AND FRESHLY GROUND PEPPER
- 75G | 2.6OZ CHORIZO, ROUGHLY SLICED
- 1 ONION, DICED
- 2 GARLIC CLOVES, DICED
- 2 TOMATOES, ROUGHLY CHOPPED
- 1 TBSP SMOKED PAPRIKA
- A LARGE PINCH OF SAFFRON (SEE TIP)
- 300G | 10.5OZ PAELLA RICE (ALTERNATIVELY USE ARBORIO RICE)
- 1.2L | 2.5PT STOCK (CHICKEN, SEAFOOD OR VEGETABLE)
- 100G | 3.5OZ FROZEN PEAS
- 6 KING PRAWNS
- 8 MUSSELS
- LEMON WEDGES, TO SERVE

STEP 1 Set your hob to a medium temperature and heat your oil in a large frying pan. While the oil heats, season the chicken thighs well with salt and pepper. Add them to the pan, frying until they are lightly browned all over.

STEP 2 Add the chorizo and continue frying for another 1-2 mins until it releases its oils. Remove the chicken and chorizo, and set aside, leaving the juices in the pan.

STEP 3 Add the diced onion to the saucepan and fry until it becomes soft and semi-translucent. Then add the garlic, chopped tomatoes, paprika and saffron, and cook for a couple of mins.

STEP 4 Return the chicken and chorizo to the saucepan, including any juices that have been released. Add the rice to the dish and allow that to fry for 1-2 mins.

STEP 5 Pour in the stock and give your dish a quick stir to ensure that all of the rice is covered with stock. Check the cooking time of your rice on its packaging, and leave it to simmer on a low heat, without stirring it.

STEP 6 Once your rice is about done, add your peas, prawns and mussels to the dish. If you want to, place a lid on top of the pan to allow the seafood to steam.

STEP 7 Once the prawns have turned pink and the mussels have opened (pick out and discard any that remain closed), you should be ready to serve. Garnish the paella with a few lemon wedges and enjoy.

Traditional paellas are cooked in a specialised paella pan, but a large, deep frying pan should suffice.

MAIN MEALS

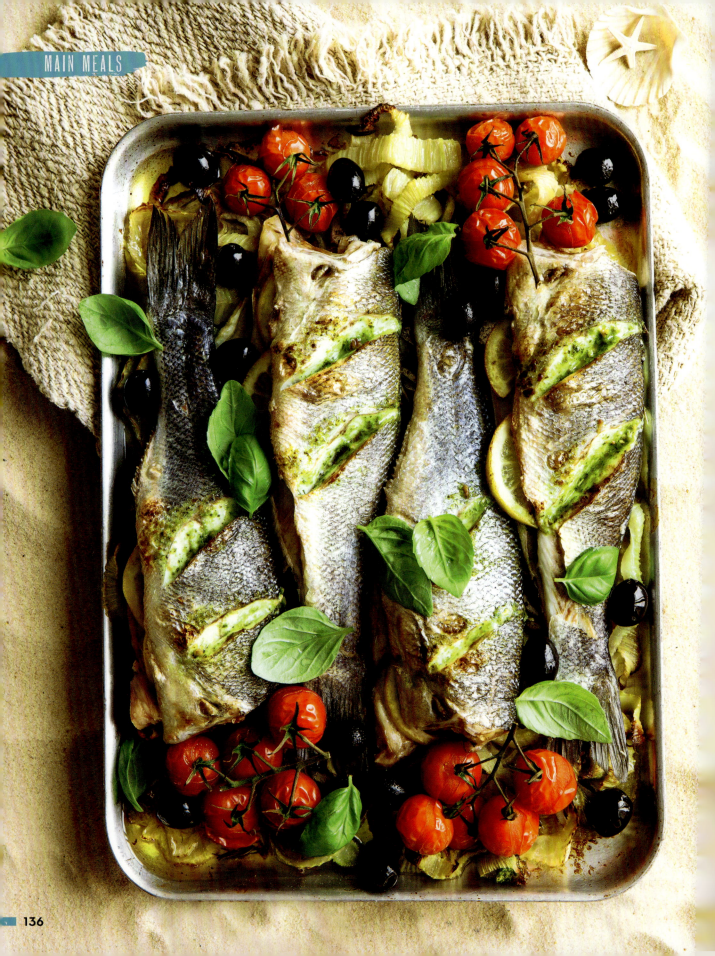

SERVINGS 4   PREP TIME 5-10 MINS   COOK TIME 25-30 MINS

MEDITERRANEAN SEA BASS BAKE

READY IN JUST OVER HALF AN HOUR, THIS IS A PERFECT QUICK MEAL

377 CALORIES

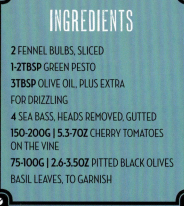

INGREDIENTS

- **2** FENNEL BULBS, SLICED
- **1-2TBSP** GREEN PESTO
- **3TBSP** OLIVE OIL, PLUS EXTRA FOR DRIZZLING
- **4** SEA BASS, HEADS REMOVED, GUTTED
- **150-200G | 5.3-7OZ** CHERRY TOMATOES ON THE VINE
- **75-100G | 2.6-3.5OZ** PITTED BLACK OLIVES
- BASIL LEAVES, TO GARNISH

STEP 1 Preheat the oven to 200°C (180°C fan) | 400°F | gas 6. Cook the fennel in boiling water for around 5-7 mins. Drain it well and spread it out in the base of a roasting tin.

STEP 2 Stir the pesto into the 3tbsp olive oil until it is evenly mixed. Slash the top flesh of the fish with a sharp knife and spoon the pesto oil in each of the slashes, then place the fish on the fennel. Drizzle over some more olive oil and bake for 10 mins.

STEP 3 Add the tomatoes (on the vine but cut into small bunches) and olives, then drizzle over a little more oil and bake for a further 10-15 mins, or until the fish is cooked.

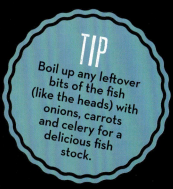

TIP
Boil up any leftover bits of the fish (like the heads) with onions, carrots and celery for a delicious fish stock.

MAIN MEALS

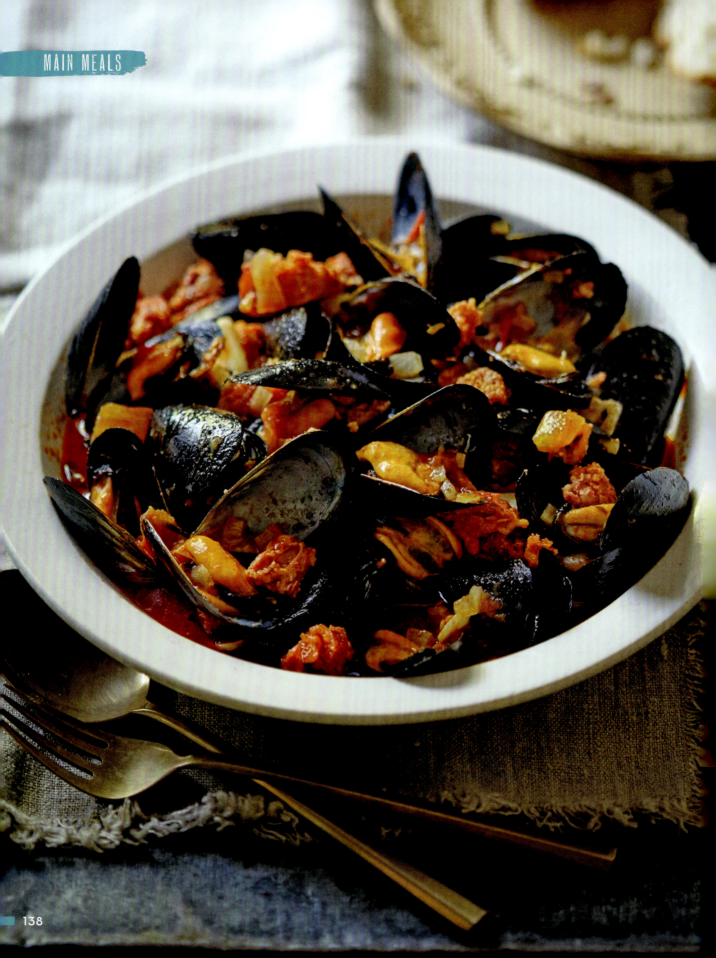

SERVINGS 2 **PREP TIME** 15 MINS **COOK TIME** 20 MINS

MUSSELS WITH CHORIZO

TAKING INSPIRATION FROM THE FLAVOURS IN SPANISH PAELLA, THIS IS A MUSSEL DISH THAT EVERYONE WILL ADORE

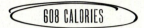
608 CALORIES

INGREDIENTS

- 4 STRANDS OF SAFFRON
- 1KG | 2.2LB MUSSELS
- 2 COOKING CHORIZO SAUSAGES (ABOUT 200G | 7OZ TOTAL), CUT INTO CHUNKS
- 1 ONION, DICED
- 2 GARLIC CLOVES, SLICED
- 2 RIPE PLUM TOMATOES, ROUGHLY CHOPPED
- 100ML | 3.4FLOZ DRY WHITE WINE
- BREAD, TO SERVE

STEP 1 Put the saffron into 25ml | 0.8floz warm water and allow it to steep for 15 mins before you begin cooking.

STEP 2 Meanwhile, thoroughly clean the mussels, removing any barnacles. Remove the beard by tugging it toward the rounded end. Tap any that are open on the edge of the sink. They should close up. Discard any that don't. Heat a large, lidded pan, then reduce the heat slightly. Add the chorizo and sizzle for 2 mins.

STEP 3 Stir in the onion, reduce the heat again and sweat, with the lid on, for 5 mins, stirring occasionally. Add the garlic and cook for 1 min until fragrant.

STEP 4 Add the tomatoes and sweat for a further 3-4 mins, until mushy. Add the wine and deglaze the sides and the pan, then bring to a boil.

STEP 5 Add the saffron and the water it was steeped in to the pan. Drain the mussels in a colander and add to the pan. With the lid on, give the pan a shake and cook for 3-5 mins or until the shells of the mussels have popped open. (Discard any that do not open at all.) Spoon the cooked mussels and chorizo chunks into bowls.

STEP 6 Let the liquid settle in the pan so you avoid any grit. Then ladle over the mussels.

MAIN MEALS

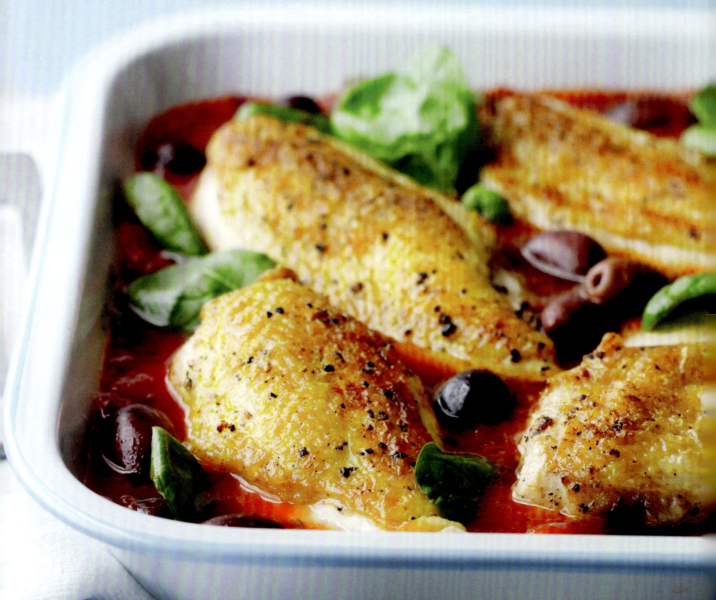

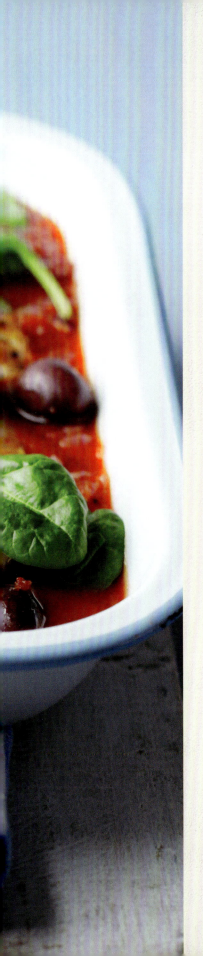

SERVINGS 4   PREP TIME 5 MINS   COOK TIME 20 MINS

MED-STYLE CHICKEN WITH BASIL AND OLIVES

EASY TO MAKE AND FULL OF FLAVOUR

308 CALORIES

INGREDIENTS

2TSP OLIVE OIL
4 CHICKEN BREASTS, SKIN ON
400G | 14.1OZ TINNED TOMATOES
1 RED ONION, FINELY CHOPPED
100ML | 3.4FLOZ CHICKEN STOCK
240G | 8.5OZ MIXED PITTED KALAMATA OLIVES, DRAINED
HANDFUL FRESH BASIL LEAVES

STEP 1 Heat the oven to 180°C (160°C fan) | 350°F | gas 6. Heat the olive oil in a pan and fry the chicken breasts, skin-side down, for 5 mins.

STEP 2 Transfer the chicken breasts to a roasting tin, skin-side up, and add the chopped tomatoes, red onion, stock and olives. Season well, then roast in the oven for 20 mins.

STEP 3 Remove the dish from the oven and scatter with the basil leaves. Serve immediately.

MAIN MEALS

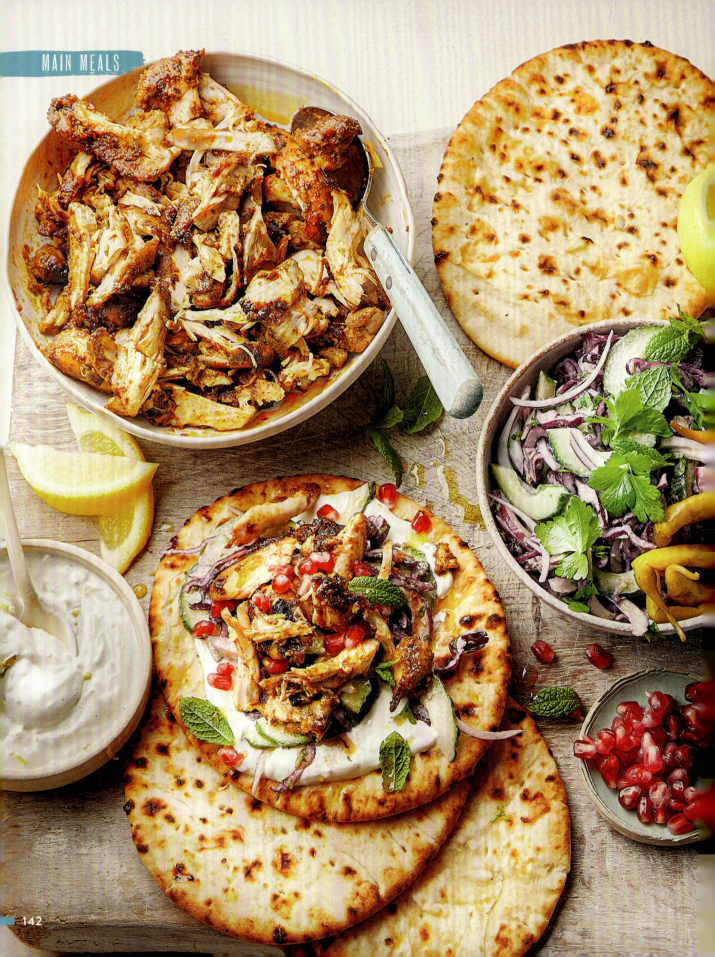

SERVINGS 4   PREP TIME 10 MINS, PLUS MARINATING   COOK TIME 35–40 MINS

CHICKEN SHAWARMA

USING A SPICE PASTE, ALONG WITH A FEW TASTY EXTRAS, MEANS THIS TURKISH WEEKEND TREAT CAN BE ON THE TABLE IN A FLASH

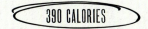
390 CALORIES

INGREDIENTS

- 8 SKINLESS, BONELESS CHICKEN THIGHS
- 4TBSP SHAWARMA PASTE (WE USED BELAZU)
- 4TBSP OLIVE OIL
- 250G | 8.8OZ GREEK YOGHURT
- 1/2 GARLIC CLOVE, CRUSHED
- 4 FLATBREADS, WARMED, TO SERVE
- SMALL HANDFUL FRESH MINT, TO SERVE
- SEEDS FROM 1/2 POMEGRANATE, TO SERVE
- PICKLED GREEN CHILLIES, TO SERVE (OPTIONAL)

FOR THE SLAW:
- 1/2 RED CABBAGE, SHREDDED
- 1/2 RED ONION, THINLY SLICED
- 1 CUCUMBER, SEEDS REMOVED AND SLICED INTO HALF MOONS
- SMALL BUNCH FRESH PARSLEY, CHOPPED (RESERVING A FEW LEAVES)
- ZEST AND JUICE 1 LEMON
- 2TBSP OLIVE OIL
- 2TBSP TAHINI

STEP 1 Put the chicken, shawarma paste, the 4tbsp olive oil and a large pinch of salt in a glass or ceramic bowl. Mix, then marinate in the fridge for at least 1 hr (or overnight).

STEP 2 Heat the oven 220°C (200°C fan) | 425°F | gas 7. Put the chicken on a baking tray and roast for 35-40 mins until slightly charred and cooked through. Remove from the oven and cool slightly before shredding.

STEP 3 Meanwhile, make the slaw. In a large bowl, mix the cabbage, red onion, cucumber and parsley. In a separate bowl, whisk together half the lemon zest, all the lemon juice, the oil, tahini and seasoning. Toss with the slaw. Set aside.

STEP 4 In a separate small bowl, mix the yoghurt, garlic and remaining lemon zest.

STEP 5 Serve the chicken, slaw and yoghurt with flatbreads, parsley, mint, pomegranate seeds and pickled chillies, if liked.

MAIN MEALS

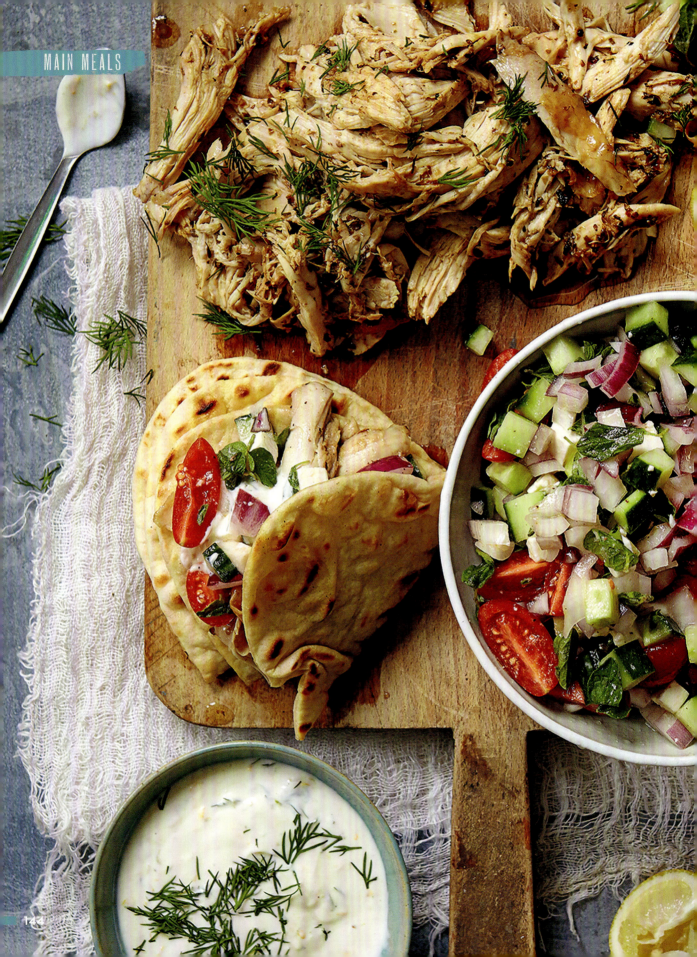

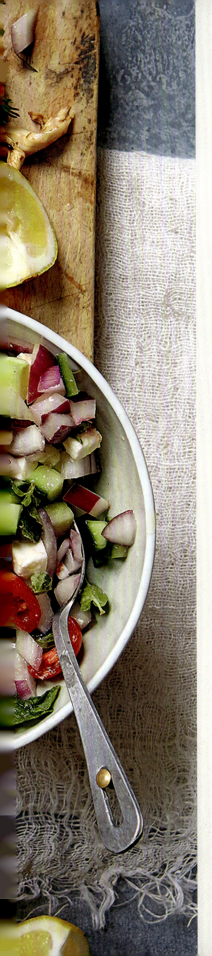

SERVINGS 4 | **PREP TIME 10 MINS, PLUS MARINATING** | **COOK TIME 1 HR 30 MINS**

GREEK ROAST CHICKEN GYROS

SPUDS AREN'T THE ONLY SIDE THAT PAIRS WELL WITH ROAST CHICKEN: THIS COMBINATION OF FLATBREAD AND SALAD MAKES A REFRESHING CHANGE WHILE STILL INDULGING OUR LOVE OF THE ROASTED BIRD

585 CALORIES

INGREDIENTS

- 6 GARLIC CLOVES, PEELED AND CRUSHED
- 2TBSP DRIED OREGANO
- 200ML | 6.8FLOZ OLIVE OIL
- JUICE AND RIND OF 1 LEMON
- 2TSP CUMIN SEEDS
- 1.5KG | 3LB WHOLE, FREE-RANGE CHICKEN
- TZATZIKI, PITTA BREADS AND GREEK SALAD TO SERVE
- A FEW DILL SPRIGS, TO SERVE

STEP 1 Preheat the oven to 180°C (160°C fan) | 350°F | gas 4. Whisk together the garlic, oregano, olive oil, lemon juice and rind and cumin seeds. Rub all over the chicken and leave to marinate in a large roasting tin for at least 15 mins or overnight.

STEP 2 Roast the chicken for 1 hr 30 mins, basting halfway, until cooked through.

STEP 3 To serve, pull the meat off the carcass and mix into the roasting juices in the pan. Let everyone make up their own pitta pockets with tzatziki and salad. Serve topped with dill.

MAIN MEALS

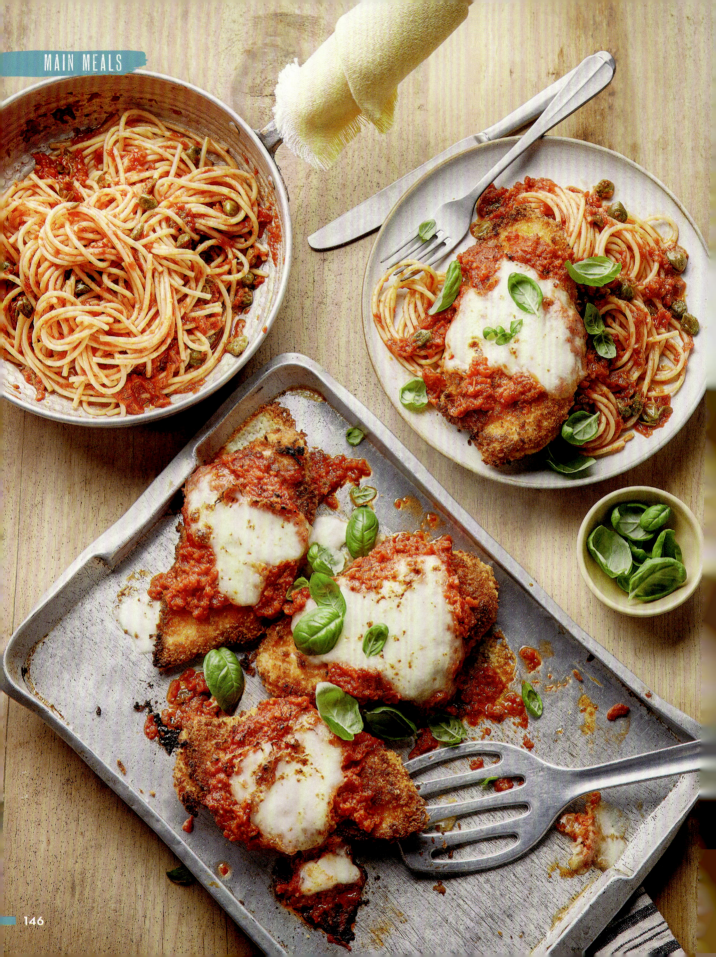

SERVINGS 4 | PREP TIME 20 MINS | COOK TIME 30 MINS

CHICKEN PARMIGIANA

CRISP CHICKEN, TANGY TOMATO SAUCE AND CHEESY TOPPING MAKE THIS CLASSIC ITALIAN DISH TOTALLY IRRESISTIBLE

831 CALORIES

INGREDIENTS

- 2 SKINLESS, BONELESS CHICKEN BREASTS, HALVED HORIZONTALLY TO MAKE 4 FILLETS
- 50G | 1.8OZ PLAIN FLOUR
- 1 MEDIUM EGG, BEATEN
- 75G | 2.6OZ PANKO BREADCRUMBS
- 30G | 1OZ PARMESAN, FINELY GRATED
- 300G | 10.6OZ SPAGHETTI
- 2TBSP VEGETABLE OIL
- 20G | 0.7OZ BUTTER
- 2X 125G | 4.4OZ BALLS MOZZARELLA, THINLY SLICED
- 4TBSP CAPERS (OPTIONAL)

FOR THE TOMATO SAUCE:
- 2TBSP OLIVE OIL
- 2 GARLIC CLOVES, CRUSHED
- 2X 400G | 14.1OZ TINS CHOPPED TOMATOES
- 1TBSP RED WINE VINEGAR
- 1TSP SMOKED PAPRIKA
- BASIL, CHOPPED, PLUS EXTRA TO GARNISH

STEP 1 Put the chicken on a board, cover with baking paper then bash with a rolling pin until it's the same thickness all over.

STEP 2 Put the flour in a dish with a pinch of salt, the egg in a second, and the breadcrumbs and half the Parmesan in a third. Dip each fillet in flour, dust off the excess, then dip in the egg and breadcrumbs. Set aside.

STEP 3 For the sauce, heat the olive oil in a saucepan, add the garlic, cook for 2 mins, then add the remaining ingredients and simmer for 10-15 mins until it thickens.

STEP 4 Heat the grill to medium. Cook the spaghetti according to pack instructions. In a large frying pan, heat the veg oil and butter, and fry the fillets for 3 mins on each side until golden. Transfer to a baking tray and top each with 1tbsp tomato sauce, the mozzarella and the remaining Parmesan. Grill until the cheese is bubbling.

STEP 5 Add the capers to the frying pan and cook on a high heat for 5 mins until crisp.

STEP 6 Stir the remaining sauce into the pasta. Serve with chicken, capers and extra basil.

MAIN MEALS

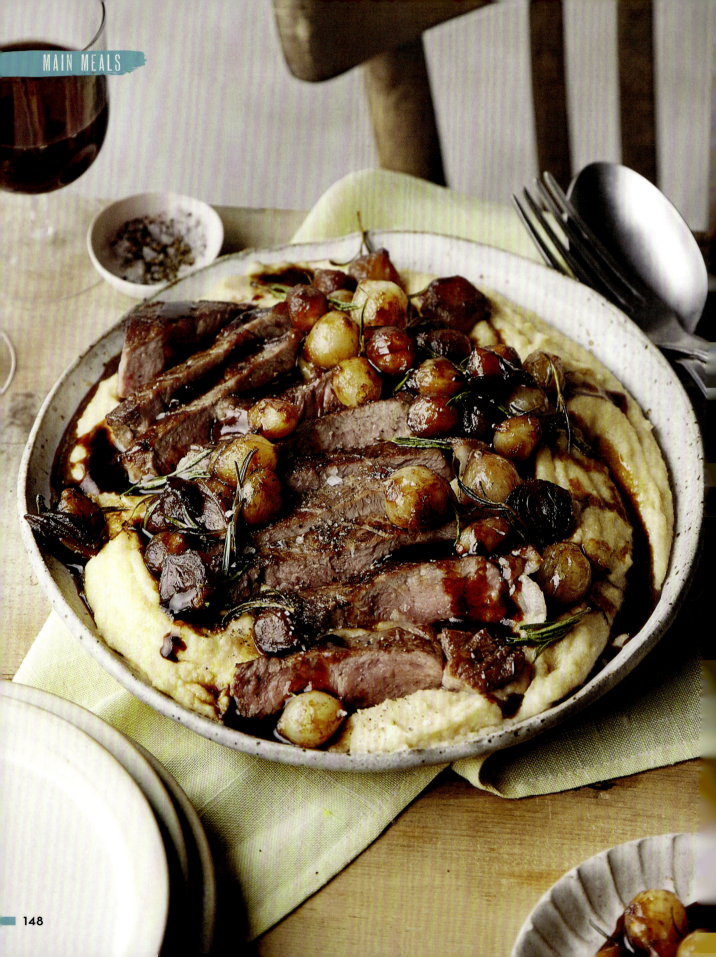

SERVINGS 4   **PREP TIME 20 MINS**   **COOK TIME 40 MINS**

VEAL STEAK WITH POLENTA

AGRODOLCE, AN ITALIAN SWEET AND SOUR SAUCE, MAKES A FLAVOURSOME TOPPING FOR THIS EASY SHARING DISH

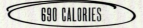
690 CALORIES

INGREDIENTS

2 THICK-CUT BRITISH ROSE VEAL STEAKS (ABOUT **250G | 8.8OZ** EACH)
1TBSP VEGETABLE OIL
KNOB OF BUTTER
SPRIG ROSEMARY

FOR THE AGRODOLCE ONIONS:
KNOB OF BUTTER
1TBSP OLIVE OIL
400G | 14.1OZ PEARL ONIONS, PEELED (WE USED FROZEN), LARGER ONES HALVED
2TBSP CASTER SUGAR
4TBSP BALSAMIC VINEGAR
SPRIG ROSEMARY, LEAVES PICKED

FOR THE POLENTA:
500ML | 16.9FLOZ CHICKEN STOCK
300ML | 10.1FLOZ WHOLE MILK
60G | 2.1OZ SALTED BUTTER
250G | 8.8OZ QUICK-COOK POLENTA
50G | 1.8OZ PARMESAN CHEESE, GRATED

STEP 1 Heat the oven to 140°C (120°C fan) | 275°F | gas 1. Pat the steaks dry and season liberally on both sides with salt. Put on a rack set over a baking tray and roast for 20 mins for medium, or up to 30 mins for well done. Set aside for 10 mins to rest.

STEP 2 Meanwhile, for the onions, melt the butter and oil in a large frying pan over medium-high heat. Add the onions and cook for 10-15 mins until golden. Stir in the sugar and balsamic vinegar and cook, stirring for 30 secs until sticky, then remove from the heat and stir in the rosemary.

STEP 3 For the polenta, put the stock, milk, half the butter and 200ml | 6.8floz water in a large saucepan. Bring to a simmer, then season well and whisk in the polenta. Cook, stirring over low heat for 3-4 mins until the polenta is cooked. Stir in the Parmesan and remaining butter.

STEP 4 Heat a large heavy frying pan (ideally cast iron) over a high heat. Brush the steaks with oil and sear both sides for 1-2 mins to form a golden crust, adding the butter and rosemary sprig halfway, and basting.

STEP 5 Spread the polenta over a warm platter. Thickly slice the steaks and arrange on top of the polenta. Stir any resting juices and herby butter from the meat into the onions and spoon over the steak. Serve with a sharply dressed leafy green salad, if liked.

MAIN MEALS

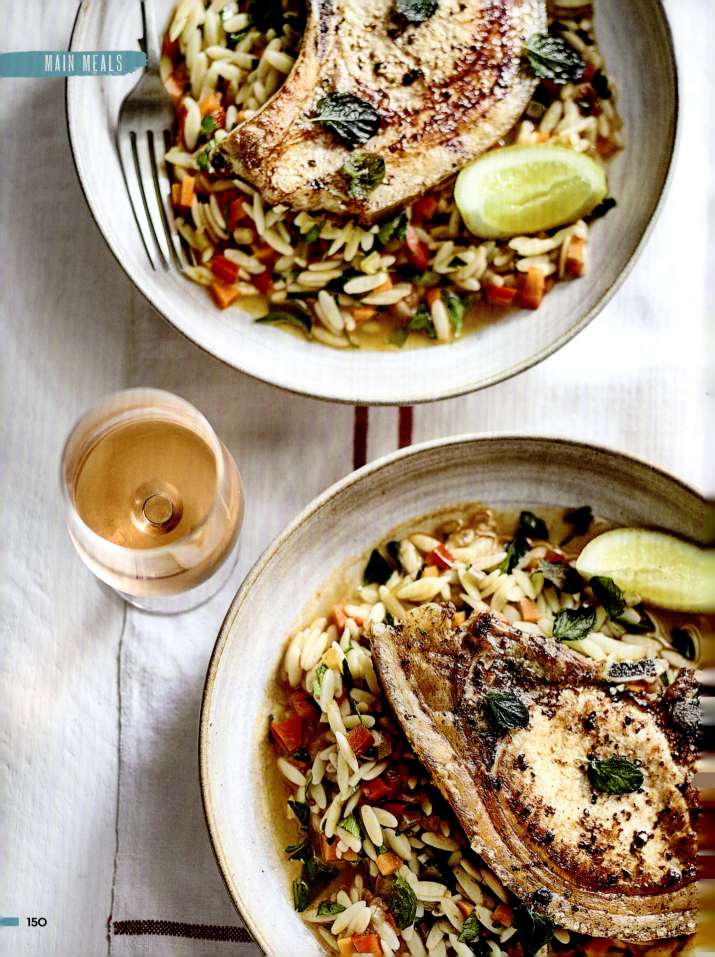

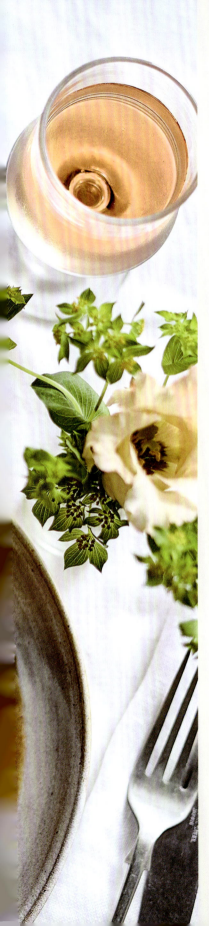

SERVINGS 4   **PREP TIME** 5 MINS   **COOK TIME** 30 MINS

PORK CHOPS WITH ORZO

A LEAN MEATY DISH WITH SIMPLE CLASSIC FLAVOURS FROM THE MED. IF YOU CAN'T FIND ORZO (RICE-SHAPED PASTA), SWAP FOR MACARONI OR BREAK UP SOME SPAGHETTI

332 CALORIES

INGREDIENTS

- 4 PORK CHOPS
- 6 FRESH OREGANO SPRIGS
- 2 TBSP OLIVE OIL
- 400G | 14.1OZ PACK FRESH OR FROZEN SOFFRITTO
- 1 RED BELL PEPPER, CHOPPED
- 3 TBSP SUN-DRIED TOMATO PASTE
- 200G | 7OZ ORZO
- 20G | 0.7 PARSLEY, LEAVES ONLY, CHOPPED
- 1 LEMON, CUT INTO 8 WEDGES

STEP 1 Heat the oven to 200°C (180°C fan) | 400°F | gas 6. Put the pork chops in a roasting tray. Scatter in the oregano sprigs, then drizzle with half the oil. Season with salt and pepper and roast the chops for 15-20 mins or until cooked through, then set aside to rest.

STEP 2 Meanwhile, heat the remaining oil in a non-stick frying pan and gently cook the soffritto mix and pepper for 10 mins. Stir in the sun-dried tomato paste and 150ml | 5floz water, then simmer for 5 mins.

STEP 3 Cook the orzo according to the pack instructions. Drain, then toss with the vegetable sauce. Season with salt and a grind of black pepper, then stir in the chopped parsley.

STEP 4 Spoon the orzo between 4 plates, top with the chops, and add lemon wedges for squeezing.

MAIN MEALS

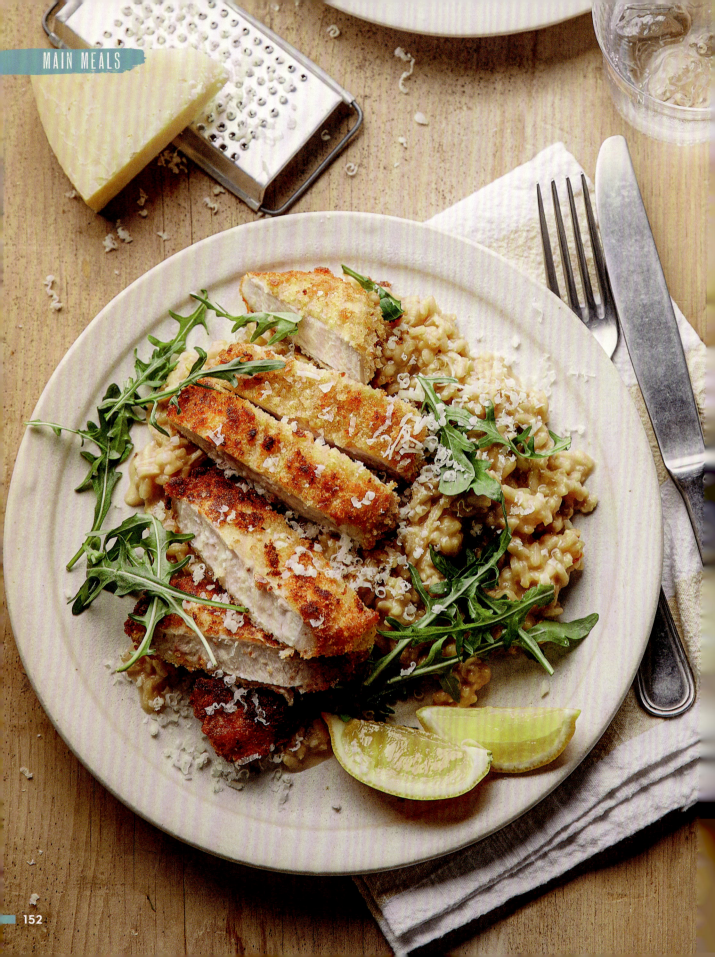

SERVINGS 4   **PREP TIME** 20 MINS   **COOK TIME** 40 MINS

PORK MILANESE WITH SAFFRON RISOTTO

THE DELICATE FLAVOUR AND GOLDEN COLOUR OF SAFFRON GIVES THIS RISOTTO A COMFORTING, EXTRA CREAMY FEEL

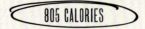
805 CALORIES

INGREDIENTS

4 BONELESS PORK CHOPS, FAT REMOVED
100G | 3.5OZ FRESH BREADCRUMBS
20G | 0.7OZ PARMESAN
2 MEDIUM EGGS, BEATEN
100G | 3.5OZ PLAIN FLOUR
VEGETABLE OIL, FOR FRYING

FOR THE RISOTTO:
1 ONION, CHOPPED
40G | 1.4OZ COLD UNSALTED BUTTER
2 LARGE GARLIC CLOVES, CRUSHED
300G | 10.6OZ ARBORIO RICE
100ML | 3.4FLOZ DRY WHITE WINE
1/2 TSP SAFFRON
1L | 2PT HOT CHICKEN STOCK
40G | 1.4OZ PARMESAN CHEESE, GRATED, PLUS EXTRA TO SERVE
1 LEMON, 1/2 ZESTED, 1/2 CUT INTO WEDGES
HANDFUL ROCKET/ARUGULA, TO SERVE

STEP 1 Cover the pork with baking paper and bash with a rolling pin until slightly flattened. Add the breadcrumbs to a plate and mix in the Parmesan. Add the eggs and flour to 2 separate plates.

STEP 2 Fry the onion in 20g | 0.7oz of the butter for 5 mins in a sauté pan. Add the garlic and cook for 1 min. Stir in the rice to coat in butter for 2-3 mins. Pour in the wine; let it bubble for 2 mins, then add the saffron.

STEP 3 Add the stock, a ladle at a time, stirring continuously, adding more as each ladleful is absorbed. Cook for 10-15 mins until the rice is starting to soften. Turn off the heat.

STEP 4 Add veg oil to a shallow pan to 1/2 way up the sides. Dip each chop in flour, egg, then breadcrumbs. Fry on a high heat for 4-5 mins, turning halfway, until crispy and cooked through. Drain on paper towels.

STEP 5 Return the risotto to the heat and stir in the remaining butter and the Parmesan. Slice the pork and place on top of the risotto. Serve with lemon zest, rocket, Parmesan and lemon wedges.

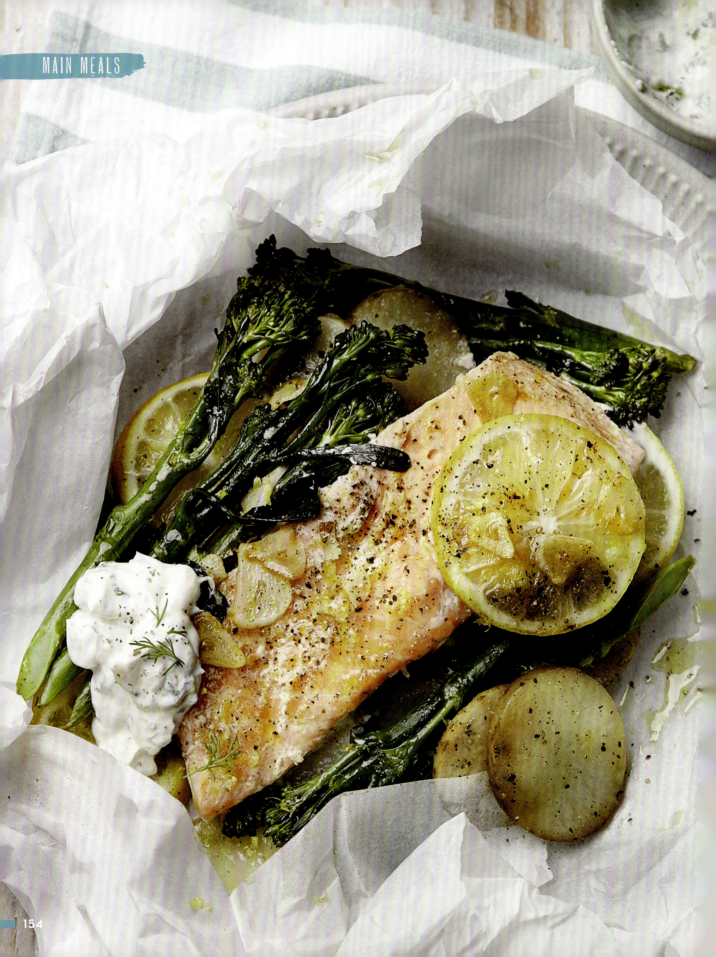

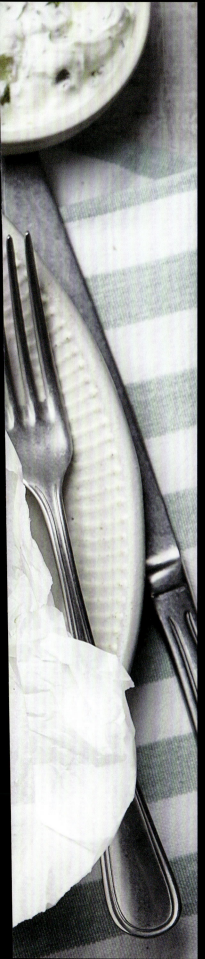

SERVINGS 1 | PREP TIME 10 MINS | COOK TIME 15-20 MINS

SALMON PARCELS

THIS EASY AND DELICIOUS MEDITERRANEAN SALMON DISH IS PACKED WITH PLENTY OF ESSENTIAL VITAMINS AND MINERALS TO HELP KEEP YOU FEELING HEALTHY

595 CALORIES

INGREDIENTS

130G | 4.6OZ NEW POTATOES
130G | 4.6OZ SALMON FILLET
1 LARGE GARLIC CLOVE, ROUGHLY CHOPPED
1TSP UNSALTED BUTTER
80G | 2.8OZ TENDERSTEM BROCCOLI/BROCCOLINI, TRIMMED
2 LEMONS, 1 ZESTED, 1 CUT INTO SLICES

FOR THE SAUCE:
50G | 1.8OZ GREEK YOGHURT
SMALL HANDFUL GHERKINS/PICKLES OR CORNICHONS, CHOPPED
SMALL BUNCH DILL
1TBSP EXTRA VIRGIN OLIVE OIL
1/2TSP WHOLEGRAIN MUSTARD

STEP 1 Heat the oven 190°C (170°C fan) | 375°F | gas 5. Parboil the potatoes for 5 mins to soften. Cool then thinly slice.

STEP 2 Cut a large square of foil, then line with baking paper. Put the salmon fillet in the middle and add the sliced potatoes, garlic, butter, broccoli, lemon slices and lemon zest. Season then wrap up tightly in the middle and around the sides, to completely seal.

STEP 3 Bake in the oven for 15-20 mins until everything is cooked and tender.

STEP 4 Meanwhile, mix all the sauce ingredients to combine.

STEP 5 Serve the salmon in its parcel (opened) with the sauce dolloped on top.

MAIN MEALS

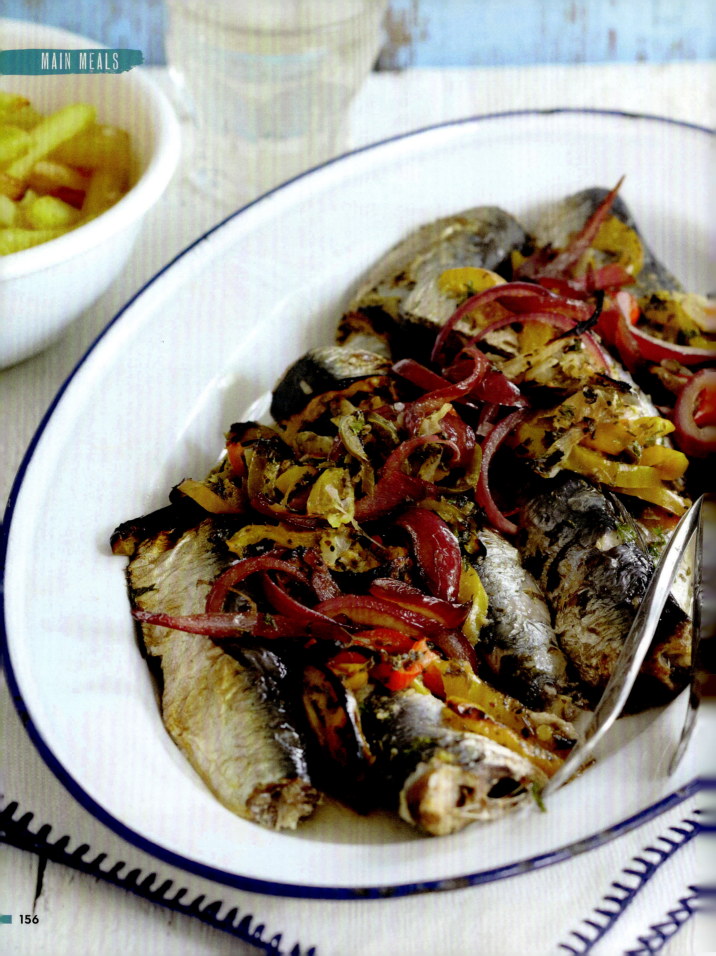

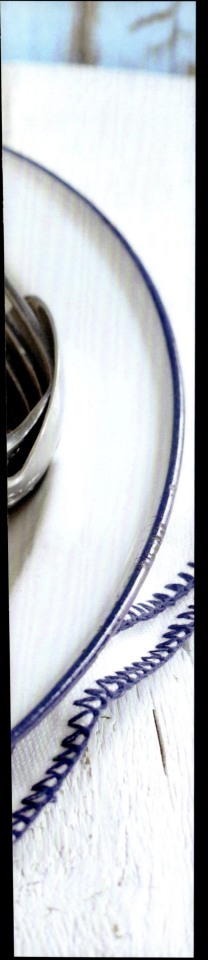

SERVINGS 4 | PREP TIME 20 MINS | COOK TIME 25 MINS

PORTUGUESE SARDINES

DELICIOUS, BUT FIDDLY. FOR EASE, ASK YOUR FISHMONGER TO PREPARE THE SARDINES, OR BUY READY-PREPARED FROM THE SUPERMARKET

483 CALORIES

INGREDIENTS

1KG | 2LB FRESH SARDINES
2 YELLOW BELL PEPPERS AND 1 RED PEPPER, THINLY SLICED
1 RED ONION, SLICED
1TBSP OLIVE OIL
2TBSP FINELY CHOPPED PARSLEY
2TBSP FINELY CHOPPED BASIL
1 GARLIC CLOVE, CRUSHED
GRATED ZEST AND JUICE OF 1 LEMON, PLUS 1 LEMON, SLICED INTO WEDGES

STEP 1 Heat the oven to 200°C (180°C fan) | 400°F | gas 6. If you're preparing the sardines, scale them by running a blunt knife from tail to head so that the scales flick off – it's best to do this in the sink. Then rinse to remove the scales and pat dry with kitchen towel. Remove the head and guts and rinse again. Pat dry, then sprinkle lightly with salt.

STEP 2 Put the peppers and onion in a roasting tin, drizzle with the oil and roast for around 20 mins until the vegetables are tender.

STEP 3 Mix the parsley and basil with the garlic, lemon zest and juice, and season lightly. Add to the vegetables and toss together.

STEP 4 Cook the sardines on a hot barbecue or under a very hot grill for 3-4 mins, turning carefully to ensure the fish don't fall apart. Put the sardines on a platter, top with the vegetables and serve with the lemon wedges.

MAIN MEALS

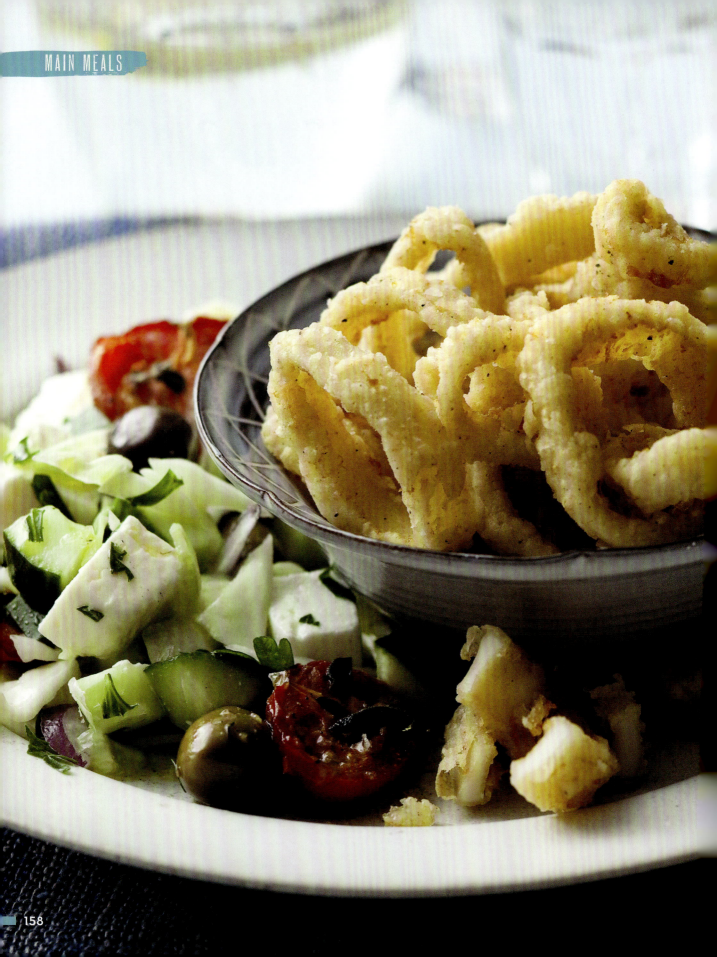

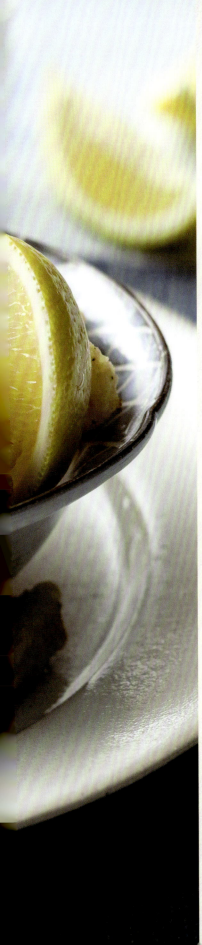

SERVINGS 4   **PREP TIME** 15 MINS   **COOK TIME** 40 MINS

FRIED SQUID

TRANSPORT YOURSELF TO A SUNNY SPANISH OR GREEK BEACH WITH THIS FLAVOURFUL CALAMARI

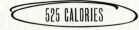

525 CALORIES

INGREDIENTS

- 8 BABY PLUM TOMATOES, HALVED
- SALT AND FRESHLY GROUND BLACK PEPPER
- 1TSP DRIED OREGANO
- 4TBSP OLIVE OIL
- 1/2 CUCUMBER, CHOPPED
- 1/2 RED ONION, THINLY SLICED
- 10 MIXED MARINATED GREEK OLIVES, DRAINED
- 1/8 WHITE CABBAGE, SHREDDED
- 200G | 7OZ GREEK FETA CHEESE, CUBED
- 2TBSP CHOPPED FRESH PARSLEY
- JUICE OF 1 LEMON
- SUNFLOWER OIL, FOR DEEP FRYING
- 4TBSP PLAIN FLOUR
- 500G | 1LB SQUID TUBES, DEFROSTED, IF FROZEN, AND SLICED
- LEMON WEDGES, TO SERVE

STEP 1 Heat the oven to 230°C (210°C fan) | 450°F | gas 8. Put the tomatoes on a roasting tray, season, sprinkle with the oregano and 2tsp oil. Roast for 10 mins. Reduce the temperature to 150°C (130°C fan) | 300°F | gas 2, and roast for 20 mins, until the tomatoes are browned around the edges but still juicy.

STEP 2 Put the cucumber, onion, olives, cabbage, feta and parsley in a bowl. Whisk the rest of the olive oil with the lemon juice, and season to taste. Pour over the salad and stir to combine. Cover and leave to allow the flavours to mingle.

STEP 3 Meanwhile, heat the sunflower oil in a deep-fat fryer to 160°C | 325°F. Put the flour on to a shallow plate and season it well. Coat the squid in the flour. Put some crumpled kitchen paper on to a tray ready to drain the squid.

STEP 4 Fry the squid in batches for a few mins, until golden. Drain on the kitchen paper.

STEP 5 Serve the roasted tomatoes with the Greek salad, squid and lemon wedges.

MAIN MEALS

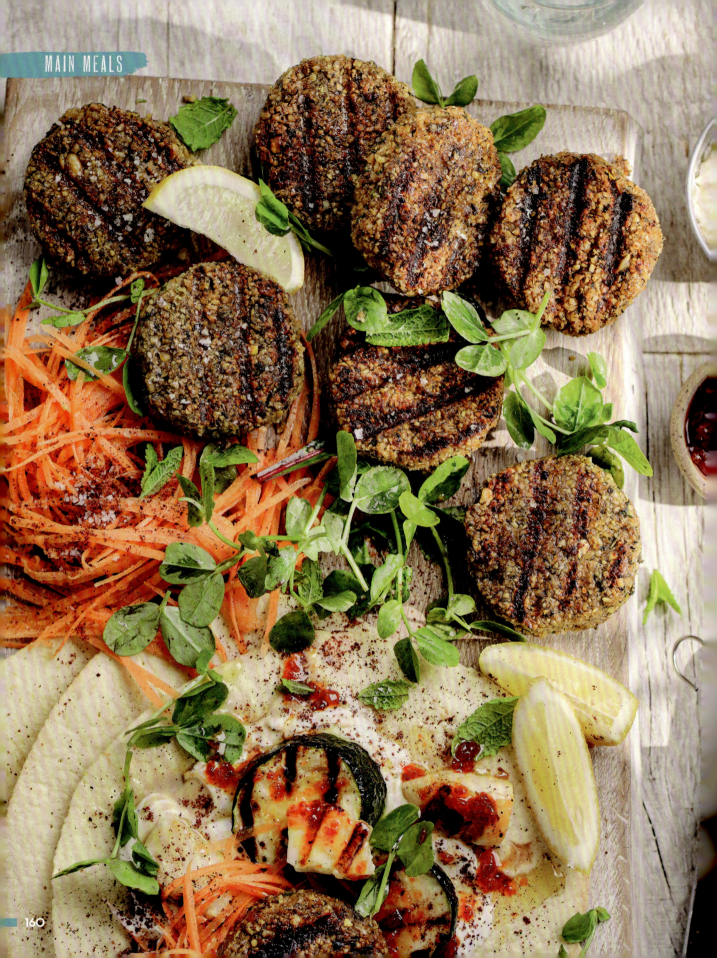

SERVINGS 4-8 **PREP TIME 20 MINS, PLUS OVERNIGHT SOAKING** **COOK TIME 10-15 MINS**

FALAFEL HALLOUMI SKEWERS

ORIGINATING IN EGYPT, FALAFELS ARE POPULAR THROUGHOUT THE MEDITERRANEAN

525 CALORIES

INGREDIENTS

- **500G | 1LB** HALLOUMI, CUT INTO 2CM | 0.8" CHUNKS
- **2** COURGETTES/ZUCCHINIS, CUT INTO 1.5CM | 0.6" CHUNKS
- **3TBSP** OLIVE OIL; EXTRA FOR BRUSHING
- **3TBSP** CHILLI JAM, LOOSENED WITH WATER
- **4TBSP** GREEK YOGHURT
- **1TBSP** TAHINI
- FLATBREADS, TOASTED, TO SERVE
- **2** LARGE CARROTS, JULIENNED OR GRATED
- **60G | 2.1OZ** BAG PEA SHOOTS
- EXTRA VIRGIN OLIVE OIL, FOR DRIZZLING
- LEMON WEDGES, FOR SQUEEZING

FOR THE FALAFEL:
- **200G | 7OZ** DRIED CHICKPEAS, SOAKED OVERNIGHT IN COLD WATER
- **2** GARLIC CLOVES, CHOPPED
- **1TBSP** BAHARAT OR LEBANESE SPICE MIX
- **1TSP** SUMAC, PLUS EXTRA TO SERVE
- **2TBSP** TAHINI
- **20G | 0.7OZ** FRESH FLAT LEAF/ITALIAN PARSLEY, 1/2 FINELY CHOPPED
- **20G | 0.7OZ** FRESH MINT, 1/2 FINELY CHOPPED
- FINELY GRATED ZEST 1/2 LEMON, JUICE
- **1 1/2-1TSP** ALL-PURPOSE SEASONING

STEP 1 First make the falafel. Drain the chickpeas and add to a food processor with the remaining ingredients and seasoning.

STEP 2 Whizz to combine, then tip into a bowl, scrunch together with your hands and shape into 8 equal-sized patties. Set aside on a lined tray and brush with oil.

STEP 3 When ready to cook, heat/light a barbecue or grill until hot.

STEP 4 In a bowl, toss halloumi and courgettes with oil and seasoning. Thread on skewers.

STEP 5 Arrange the falafel on the grill and cook for 8-10 mins, turning. Place the halloumi skewers around the edge. Grill for 5 mins, turning regularly until charred and tender, then, off the grill, brush with the chilli jam.

STEP 6 Serve the falafel and skewers with the Greek yoghurt mixed with the tahini, plus flatbreads, carrots, pea shoots, a drizzle of oil and lemon wedges for squeezing. Sprinkle the carrot and salad with sumac.

DESSERTS

Tarta di Santiago	165
Churros with salted caramel affogato	167
Gelo di melone	169
Crostata di pistachio con ricotta e limone tart	171
Pasteis de nata	173
Tiramisu	175
Kremsnita	177
Pistachio baklava	179
Crème brûlée	181
Lemon sorbet	183
Crème caramel	185
Basque-style burnt cheesecake with honey roasted figs	187
Latte panna cotta	189
Poached pears with fresh ricotta, honey and pine nuts	191
Pistachio, rose and olive oil cake	193
Orange polenta cake	195

DESSERTS

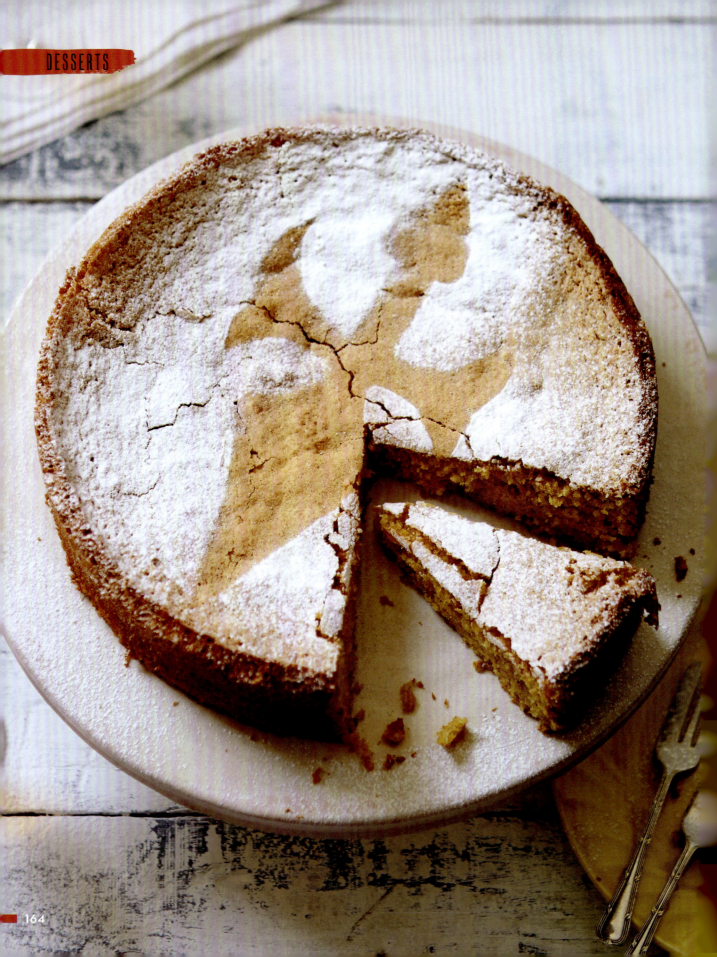

SERVINGS 8 | **PREP TIME** 10 MINS | **REST TIME** 10 MINS | **COOK TIME** 40-45 MINS

TARTA DI SANTIAGO

THIS TRADITIONAL SPANISH ALMOND CAKE IS NATURALLY GLUTEN-FREE AND MADE WITHOUT BUTTER

380 CALORIES

INGREDIENTS

- 5 EGGS
- 220G | 7.8OZ CASTER SUGAR
- 250G | 8.8OZ GROUND ALMONDS
- 5 LEMONS, ZEST ONLY
- ½ TSP GROUND CINNAMON
- ICING SUGAR, TO DUST
- 25G | 0.9OZ ROUGHLY CHOPPED ALMONDS, TO SERVE
- GREEK YOGHURT, TO SERVE

YOU WILL NEED:
23CM | 9" SPRINGFORM CAKE TIN, GREASED AND LINED WITH BAKING PAPER
A PIECE OF PAPER TO CUT OUT AS A STENCIL (OPTIONAL)

STEP 1 Preheat the oven to 180°C (160°C fan) | 355°F | gas 4. Put the eggs and sugar in a bowl and whisk them together until thick and pale. Fold in the ground almonds, lemon zest and cinnamon.

STEP 2 Pour the mixture into the cake tin and bake for 40-45 mins or until a skewer inserted in the middle comes out clean. Set the tin on a wire rack for 10 mins before removing the cake from the tin.

STEP 3 Once the cake is cool, put the template on top (if using) and dust over the icing sugar. Serve with the chopped almonds and a dollop of Greek yoghurt.

TIP

You don't have to use the traditional stencil shape – feel free to cut out any shape you like.

THIS CAKE ORIGINATES FROM GALICIA DURING TIMES OF MEDIEVAL PILGRIMAGES, WHICH IS WHY IT IS TRADITIONALLY DECORATED WITH THE ST JAMES' CROSS.

DESSERTS

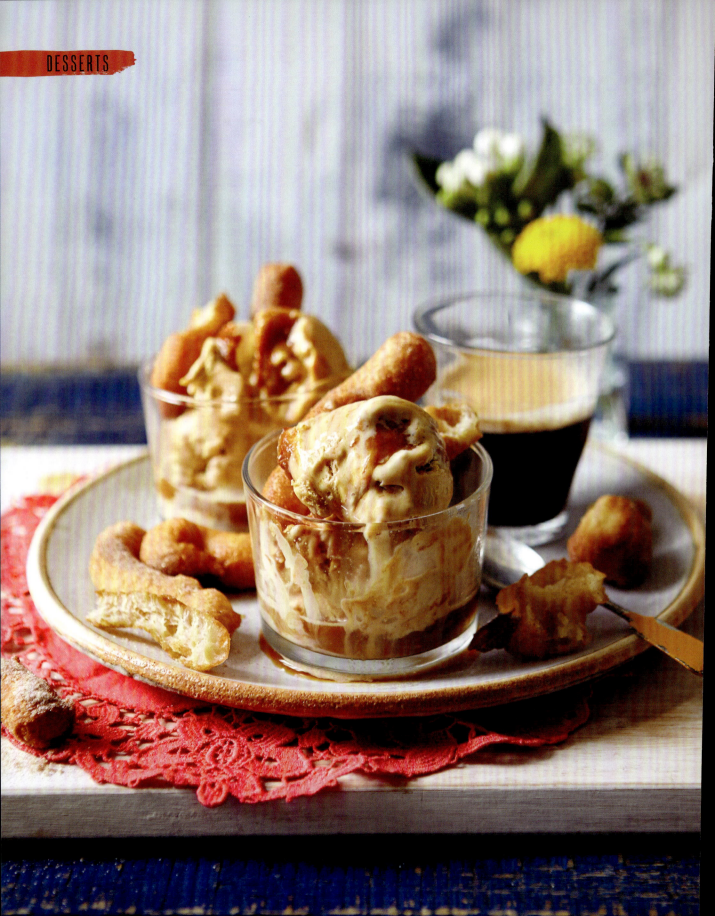

SERVINGS 4 | PREP TIME 5-10 MINS | CHILL TIME 30 MINS | COOK TIME 10-15 MINS

CHURROS WITH SALTED CARAMEL AFFOGATO

THESE SPANISH DOUGHNUTS ARE PERFECT WITH AFFOGATO, AN ITALIAN DESSERT OF ICE CREAM WITH A HOT ESPRESSO COFFEE POURED OVER IT

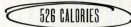
526 CALORIES

INGREDIENTS

1TBSP OLIVE OIL, PLUS PLENTY MORE FOR DEEP FRYING
1TSP VANILLA EXTRACT
250G | 8.8OZ PLAIN FLOUR, SIFTED
1TBSP BAKING POWDER
1TSP GROUND CINNAMON
2TBSP CASTER SUGAR
4 SCOOPS SALTED CARAMEL ICE CREAM
4 CUPS HOT STRONG COFFEE, TO SERVE

YOU WILL NEED:
PIPING BAG WITH A 1CM | 0.4" STAR-SHAPED NOZZLE

STEP 1 For the churros, bring 200ml | 6.8floz water to the boil in a large saucepan with the 1tbsp olive oil and vanilla. Add the flour and baking powder and stir well until you have a thick paste. Remove from the heat and leave to cool.

STEP 2 Put the dough in a piping bag and chill in the freezer for 30 mins. Pour the olive oil into a deep-fat fryer or heavy-based saucepan to a depth of 10cm | 4". Heat the oil to 160°C | 320°F (use a sugar thermometer or drop a cube of bread into the oil – when it turns golden within 1 min, it is the right temperature).

STEP 3 Very carefully pipe 10cm | 4" lengths of the dough into the oil, using scissors to snip off the ends. Fry the churros for 3-4 mins, turning if necessary, until golden. Remove from the oil with a slotted spoon and drain on kitchen paper.

STEP 4 Mix the cinnamon and sugar, then dust over the churros while still warm. Spoon ice cream into glass coffee cups. Pour over the coffee and serve immediately with a few churros.

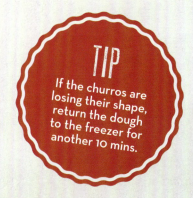

TIP
If the churros are losing their shape, return the dough to the freezer for another 10 mins.

DESSERTS

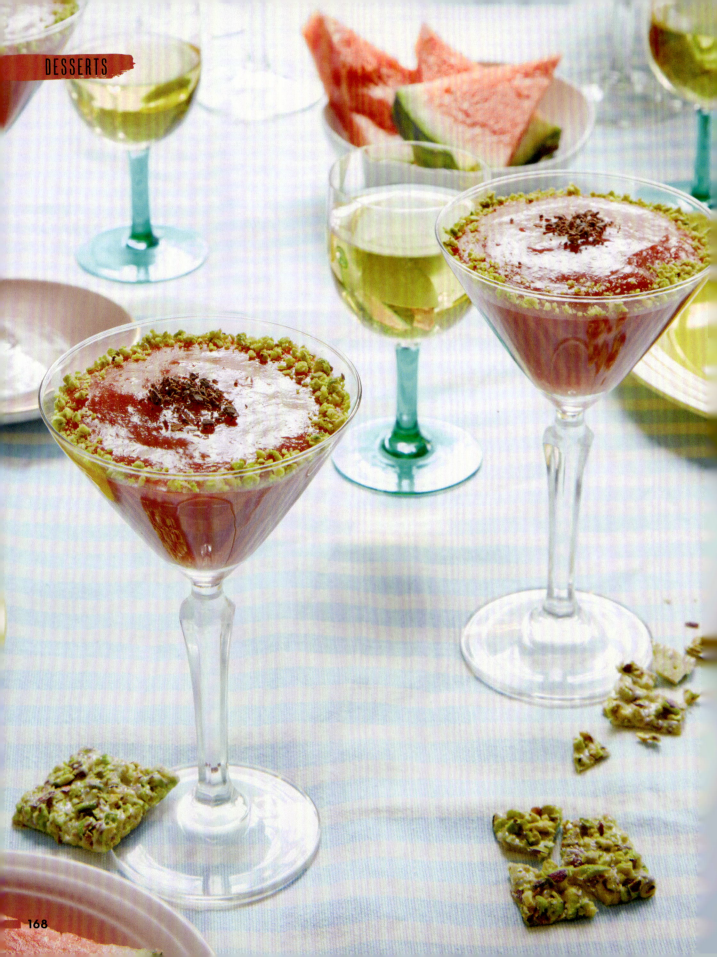

SERVINGS 6 | **PREP TIME 10-15 MINS** | **CHILL TIME 2 HRS** | **COOK TIME 15 MINS**

GELO DI MELONE

THIS JOYFULLY WOBBLY DESSERT IS HALF PUDDING, HALF JELLY AND HAILS FROM SICILY'S CAPITAL, PALERMO

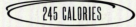

245 CALORIES

INGREDIENTS

- 100G | 3.5OZ CORNFLOUR/CORNSTARCH
- 1L | 2 PT WATERMELON JUICE (SEE TIP)
- 100G | 3.5OZ CASTER SUGAR
- ¼TSP GROUND CINNAMON, PLUS EXTRA FOR DECORATING
- 50G | 1.8OZ PISTACHIO NUTS, TO SERVE
- 40G | 1.4OZ DARK/BITTERSWEET CHOCOLATE, SHAVED, TO SERVE

STEP 1 In a large saucepan over a moderate heat, whisk the cornflour with 250ml | 8.5floz watermelon juice, mixing well to make sure there are no lumps.

STEP 2 Add the rest of the watermelon juice, sugar and cinnamon, and bring to a simmer, whisking constantly to ensure no lumps form.

STEP 3 Simmer for around 10 mins until the mixture has thickened and coats the back of a spoon. Pour into glasses or ramekins and chill in the fridge for at least 2 hrs.

STEP 4 Blitz three-quarters of the pistachios in a food processor and leave the remaining ones whole for texture. Before serving, top the desserts with the pistachios, chocolate shavings and a sprinkling of cinnamon.

TIP
To make watermelon juice, blitz 800g | 28.2oz watermelon chunks in a blender and pass it through a sieve.

Palermo chefs devised the recipe to use up watermelons at the end of summer.

DESSERTS

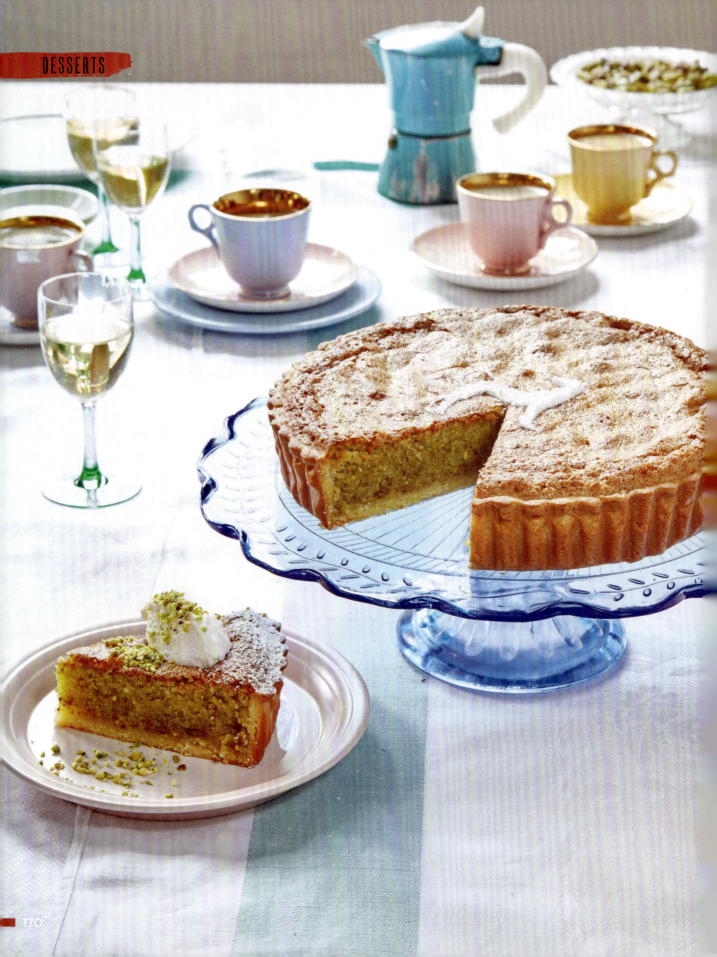

SERVINGS 8 | PREP TIME 20 MINS | CHILL TIME 35-45 MINS | COOK TIME 35-40 MINS

CROSTATA DI PISTACHIO CON RICOTTA E LIMONE TART

THIS RICH, NUTTY DESSERT IS A SPECIALITY OF SICILIAN CHEF EMILIA STRAZZANTI, WHO HAS KINDLY SHARED HER PRIZED RECIPE

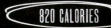

820 CALORIES

INGREDIENTS

FOR THE PASTRY:
- 105ML | 3.6FLOZ OLIVE OIL
- 120G | 4.2OZ CASTER SUGAR
- 4 EGG YOLKS
- 300G | 10.5OZ PLAIN FLOUR

FOR THE FILLING:
- 180ML | 6FLOZ OLIVE OIL
- 240G | 8.5OZ CASTER SUGAR
- 4 EGGS
- 80G | 2.8OZ GROUND ALMONDS
- 160G | 5.6OZ PISTACHIOS, BLITZED TO A POWDER

FOR THE RICOTTA TOPPING:
- 250G | 8.8OZ RICOTTA
- 1 LEMON, ZEST ONLY
- 150G | 5.3OZ ICING SUGAR, PLUS EXTRA TO DUST

YOU WILL NEED:
- 20CM | 8" SPRINGFORM FLAN TIN, WITH REMOVABLE BASE

STEP 1 For the pastry, beat the olive oil and sugar with an electric mixer until creamy. Add the yolks one by one, then the flour, mixing until combined. If you find the pastry is too dry, add more oil ½tsp at a time until it comes together. If it is too wet to handle, add more flour 2tsp at a time.

STEP 2 Roll out the pastry between 2 pieces of floured baking parchment to 5mm | 0.2" and line the flan tin, pushing the pastry into the corners. Cover with cling film and chill for 15 mins.

STEP 3 Meanwhile, for the filling, cream the olive oil and sugar until light and fluffy. Add the eggs one by one, mixing well after each addition, then stir in the almonds and pistachios. Mix well and pour into the pastry case. Place back into the fridge for 20-30 mins to chill slightly and preheat the oven to 170°C (150°C fan) | 340°F | gas 3.

STEP 4 Bake for 35-40 mins. Beat together the ricotta cheese, zest and icing sugar. Serve the tart dusted with icing sugar and top with a spoonful of cheese mixture.

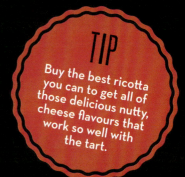

TIP
Buy the best ricotta you can to get all of those delicious nutty, cheese flavours that work so well with the tart.

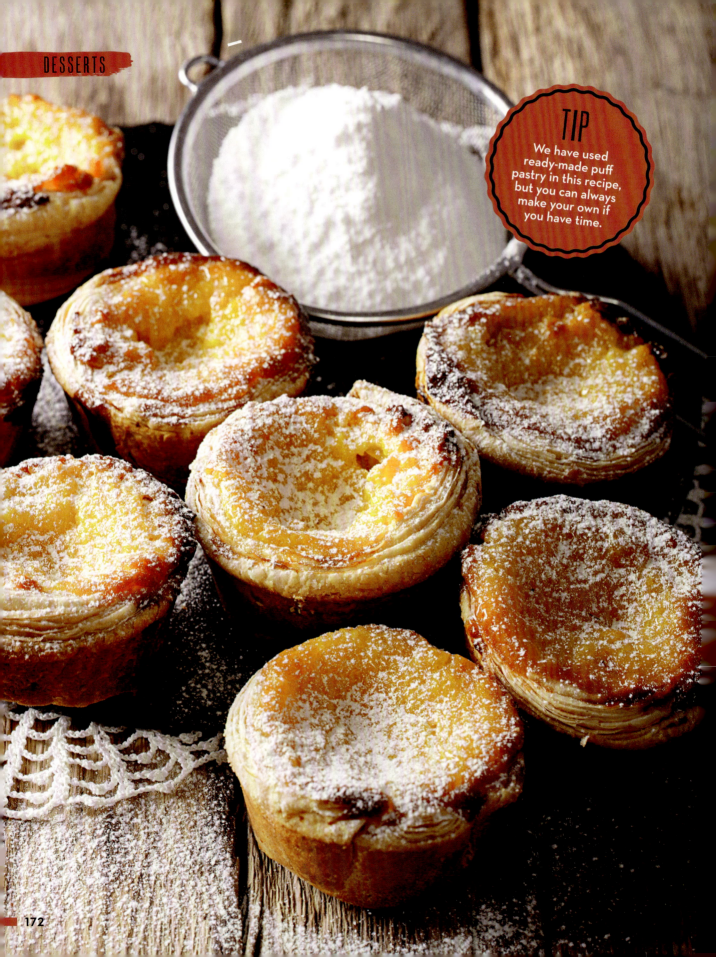

DESSERTS

TIP
We have used ready-made puff pastry in this recipe, but you can always make your own if you have time.

MAKES 30-40 TARTS | **PREP TIME 25-30 MINS** | **CHILL TIME OVERNIGHT, PLUS 15 MINS** | **COOK TIME 35-45 MINS**

PASTEIS DE NATA

TAKE YOUR TEA OR COFFEE WITH ONE OF THESE BITE-SIZED PORTUGUESE TREATS, THE ORIGINAL CUSTARD TART

285-214 CALORIES PER TART

INGREDIENTS

700G | 24.7OZ READY-ROLLED PUFF PASTRY
OLIVE OIL, FOR BRUSHING AND GREASING
4-5TBSP ICING SUGAR, FOR DUSTING
1/2-1TBSP GROUND CINNAMON (OPTIONAL)

FOR THE CUSTARD:
475ML | 16FLOZ DOUBLE/HEAVY CREAM
360ML | 12.2FLOZ FULL-FAT/WHOLE MILK
1 VANILLA POD, SEEDS SCRAPED (OR 2TSP VANILLA EXTRACT)
4TBSP CORNFLOUR/CORNSTARCH, SIFTED
225G | 8OZ CASTER SUGAR
2 LARGE EGGS
4 LARGE EGG YOLKS

YOU WILL NEED:
A MUFFIN OR CUPCAKE TIN, WITH THE WELLS GREASED (IDEALLY MULTIPLE TINS TO BAKE 30-40 PASTRIES AT ONCE)

STEP 1 Start by preparing the custard. In a large saucepan over a medium heat, add the cream, milk, and vanilla pod and seeds. Cook for 10 mins, stirring frequently. Take off the heat to cool slightly.

STEP 2 In a large bowl, sift together the cornflour and sugar. Whisk the eggs and egg yolks into this mixture to form a paste. Add 100ml | 3½floz of the hot milk mix to the egg mix, whisking constantly so the eggs don't scramble.

STEP 3 Pour the egg mixture into the saucepan with the rest of the milk, and return to the heat for another 10 mins or so. Keep whisking as the cornflour thickens the custard; it should be thick but pourable. Pass the custard through a sieve, place into a glass bowl, and cover with cling film (with the wrap in contact with the custard). Refrigerate overnight.

STEP 4 Preheat the oven to 250°C (230°C fan) | 480°F | gas 9. Unroll the pastry from its packaging and brush the top with a little olive oil. With the short edge of the pastry facing you, tightly re-roll the pastry into a log shape (repeat if you are using multiple packets of pastry). Trim the edges of the logs so they are neat, then slice them into even rounds to create about 30-40 pastry discs in total.

STEP 5 Place one pastry disc into each well of the muffin or cupcake tin. Use your fingers to press and shape the dough so it completely covers the bottom and sides of the well. The pastry should stick up a little from the top of the well, because the pastry will shrink as it bakes. Put the cases in the fridge to chill for 15 mins.

STEP 6 Pour the custard into the pastry cups until they are about ¾ full. Bake on the top shelf of the oven for 10-15 mins. Check how brown they are and bake for a further 5-10 mins if desired. The custard should have some dark-brown spots on its surface.

STEP 7 Allow to cool slightly before dusting with icing sugar and cinnamon (if using). Serve warm. The cooled pastéis can also be frozen for when you need them – simply defrost and reheat in the oven for a few mins until completely warmed through.

DESSERTS

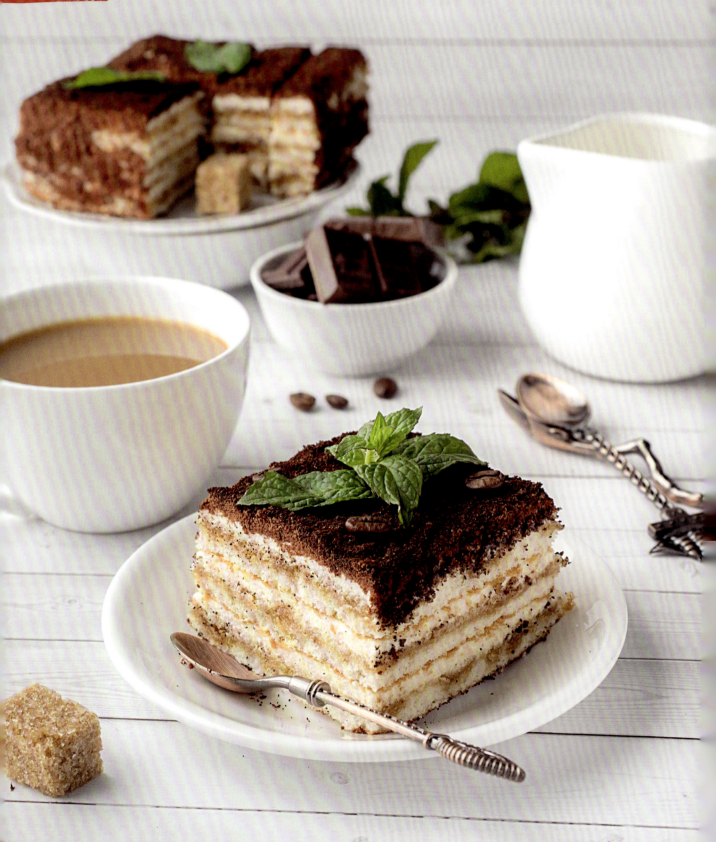

SERVINGS 8 · PREP TIME 30 MINS · CHILL TIME 4 HRS - OVERNIGHT

TIRAMISU

THIS CREAMY, COFFEE-FLAVOURED DESSERT IS THE PERFECT TREAT AT THE END OF AN ITALIAN FEAST

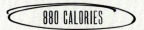
880 CALORIES

INGREDIENTS

- 200ML | 6.8FLOZ ESPRESSO COFFEE, COOLED
- 150ML | 5FLOZ MARSALA WINE, OR COFFEE LIQUEUR
- 6 EGGS, YOLKS AND WHITES SEPARATED
- 1TSP VANILLA EXTRACT
- 250G | 8.8OZ ICING SUGAR, SIFTED
- 250ML | 8.5FLOZ DOUBLE/HEAVY CREAM
- 250G | 8.8OZ FULL-FAT MASCARPONE CHEESE
- 30-36 SAVOIARDI BISCUITS (LADYFINGERS OR SPONGE FINGERS), GIVE OR TAKE A FEW DEPENDING ON THE SIZE OF THE DISH
- 3-5TBSP GRATED DARK/BITTERSWEET CHOCOLATE, OR COCOA POWDER, TO DUST
- 8 SMALL SPRIGS FRESH MINT, TO GARNISH
- 1-2TBSP WHOLE, ROASTED COFFEE BEANS, TO GARNISH

STEP 1 In a shallow bowl, combine the cooled coffee and liqueur/Marsala wine, and set aside.

STEP 2 Whisk together the egg yolks, vanilla extract and the icing sugar until the mixture is a pale-yellow colour.

STEP 3 Whisk the double cream until it stiffens and becomes spreadable. Then add the mascarpone and combine.

STEP 4 Add the sugary egg yolks into the mascarpone mix, and whisk again until the mixture is thick and thoroughly combined.

STEP 5 In another bowl, and using a clean whisk, whip the egg whites to stiff peaks. Gently fold the egg whites into the large bowl with the mascarpone mix.

STEP 6 Take the Savoiardi biscuits and – one at a time – dip them into the coffee mixture for a few seconds on each side, then place them in the bottom of a square dish. Do this until you've arranged 10-12 Savoiardi biscuits evenly in the tray.

STEP 7 Spread around one third of the mascarpone mix on top of the soaked biscuits, smoothing it over evenly.

STEP 8 Repeat step 6, placing the biscuits on top of the layer of mascarpone.

STEP 9 Repeat step 7, then repeat step 6 once again.

STEP 10 Spread the remaining mascarpone evenly over the third layer of soaked Savoiardi biscuits. Put it in the fridge to set for at least 4 hrs, or overnight.

STEP 11 Dust liberally with grated dark chocolate, and decorate with a few sprigs of fresh mint and coffee beans before serving.

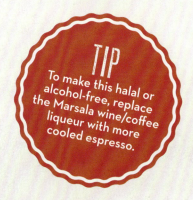
TIP To make this halal or alcohol-free, replace the Marsala wine/coffee liqueur with more cooled espresso.

DESSERTS

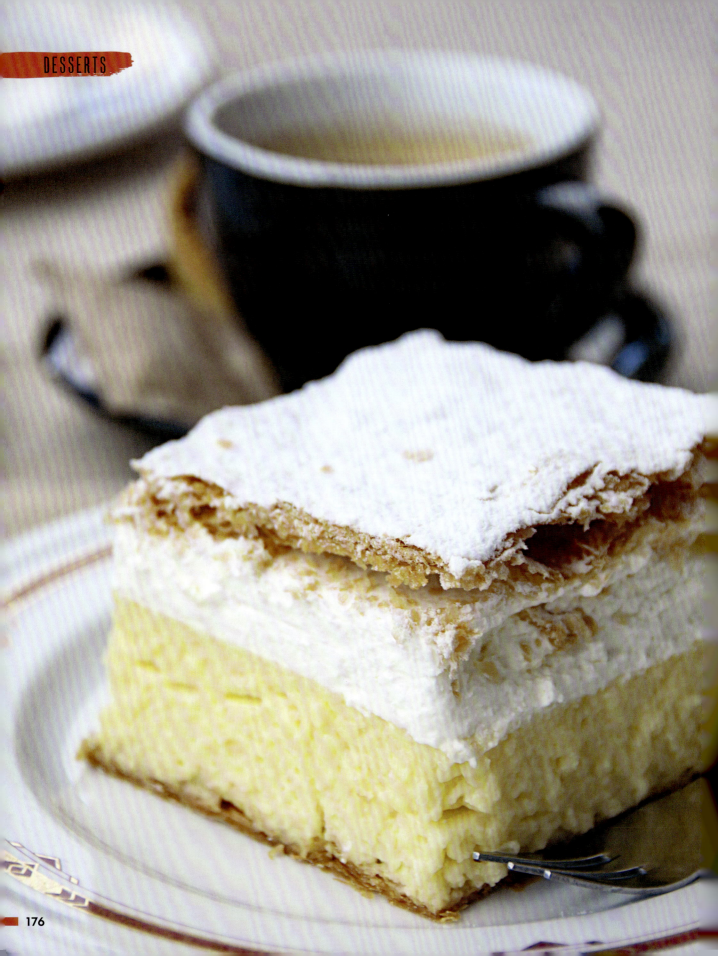

SERVINGS 9 | PREP TIME 1 HR | COOK TIME 15 MINS

KREMSNITA

A FINGER-LICKING CREAMY DESSERT FROM SLOVENIA

880 CALORIES

INGREDIENTS

500G | 17.6OZ PUFF PASTRY
2-3TBSP ICING SUGAR, FOR DUSTING

FOR THE CUSTARD:
10 EGGS
400G | 14OZ CASTER SUGAR
1.6L | 3.4PT MILK
180G | 6.3OZ PLAIN FLOUR
2TBSP VANILLA SUGAR
1TSP RUM

FOR THE VANILLA CREAM:
500ML | 17FLOZ DOUBLE/HEAVY CREAM
2TBSP ICING SUGAR
1TSP VANILLA ESSENCE

STEP 1 Roll the pastry out to the size of a large baking tray. Place it onto a prepared tray, lined with baking paper. Now prick the pastry all over with a fork and cut down the middle with a sharp knife to create two rectangles.

STEP 2 Bake the pastry in a preheated oven for 10-15 mins at 200°C (180°C fan) | 400°F | gas 6 or until golden in colour. Remove from the oven and leave it to cool while you prepare the rest.

STEP 3 Separate the egg whites and yolks, then whisk the whites with 100g | 3.5oz of caster sugar until stiff peaks form. Set aside.

STEP 4 Now whisk the egg yolks with 300g | 10.5oz of caster sugar until they begin to lighten in colour. Gently add 180ml | 6floz of the cold milk, then sift in the flour.

STEP 5 Boil the rest of the milk with the vanilla sugar, then slowly add the egg yolks, stirring as you do. Whisk over the heat for around 10 mins – the mix will thicken.

STEP 6 Slowly add the custard to the egg whites, carefully folding so as not to lose too much air. Gently stir in the rum.

STEP 7 While the mix is still warm, spread it over one of the rectangles of pastry and leave it to cool.

STEP 8 Whisk the double cream with the icing sugar and vanilla essence until it thickens. Stop when it just begins to hold its shape. Spread the cream over the top of the cooled custard followed by the other sheet of pasty and dust generously with icing sugar.

STEP 9 Chill in the fridge until firm, then slice into 9 portions.

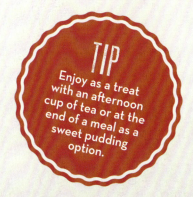

TIP Enjoy as a treat with an afternoon cup of tea or at the end of a meal as a sweet pudding option.

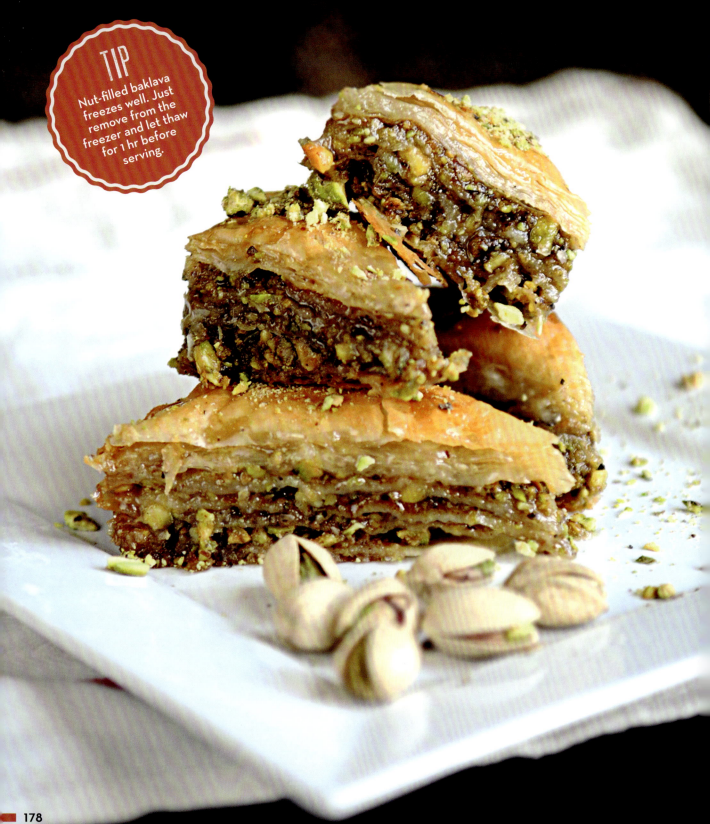

DESSERTS

TIP
Nut-filled baklava freezes well. Just remove from the freezer and let thaw for 1 hr before serving.

MAKES 25 PIECES | PREP TIME 40 MINS | REST TIME 7 HRS | COOK TIME 1 HR

PISTACHIO BAKLAVA

THESE BITE-SIZED SYRUPY FILO PASTRY MORSELS ARE A RICH AND DECADENT END TO ANY MEAL, OR A SWEET ACCOMPANIMENT TO AFTERNOON TEA

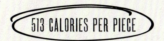

513 CALORIES PER PIECE

INGREDIENTS

FOR THE SYRUP:
- 450G | 16OZ GRANULATED SUGAR
- 425ML | 14.4FLOZ WATER
- 4TBSP HONEY
- 2 CARDAMOM PODS
- 1TBSP FRESH LEMON JUICE
- 1TSP ORANGE BLOSSOM WATER

FOR THE BAKLAVA:
- 500G | 17.6OZ PISTACHIO NUTS, COARSELY GROUND
- 60G | 2OZ GRANULATED SUGAR
- 2TSP GROUND CARDAMOM
- ½ TSP GROUND CINNAMON
- 40 SHEETS FILO PASTRY
- OLIVE OIL, FOR GREASING AND BRUSHING

STEP 1 First, prepare the syrup. In a saucepan, combine all of the ingredients. Place on a high heat, stirring frequently, and bring to the boil. Reduce to a medium heat and simmer for 20 mins.

STEP 2 To check if the syrup is ready, place a drop on a flat plate. If the drop holds its shape as the plate is tilted, then it's ready. Remove from the heat and add the orange blossom water. Mix well, then let it cool completely (about 4 hrs). Remove the cardamom pods.

STEP 3 Now prepare the baklava. Coarsely grind the pistachio nuts and set 1tbsp aside for decoration at the end. Mix the rest of the nuts in a bowl with the sugar, cardamom and cinnamon. Set aside.

STEP 4 Trim the pastry sheets to fit a baking tray (33x22cm | 13x9") and place the sheets underneath a damp towel until ready to use. Preheat the oven to 175°C (155°C fan) | 350°F | gas 4. Grease a baking tray with some olive oil.

STEP 5 Line the pan with the first pastry sheet, then brush gently with olive oil. Repeat, layering and brushing until you have 12 layers. Spread one-third of the filling over the top sheet. Then layer and brush 8 more sheets with olive oil.

STEP 6 Spread another one-third of the filling over the top sheet. Then layer and brush 8 more sheets with olive oil. Spread the final third of the filling over the top sheet. Then layer and brush 12 more sheets with olive oil.

STEP 7 Gently press the layers down and tuck in the pastry around the edges of the pan. Brush the surface with olive oil. With a sharp knife, cut into small triangles, being careful to cut all the way down to the bottom of the pan.

STEP 8 Spray the surface lightly with water, then bake in the preheated oven for 30 mins. Reduce the oven temperature to 150°C (130°C fan) | 300°F | gas 2 and continue to bake the baklava for another 30 mins, or until golden brown.

STEP 9 Remove the baklava from the oven and pour the cooled syrup over the surface. Let it sit for at least 3 hrs, then scatter the leftover ground pistachios over it to serve.

DESSERTS

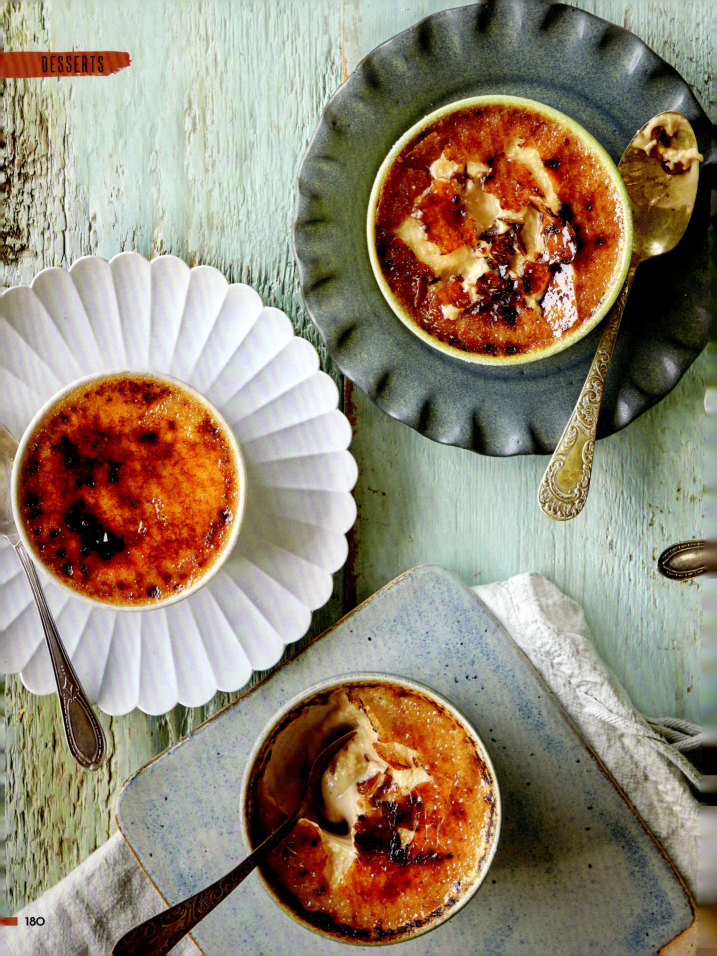

SERVINGS 8 | **PREP TIME** 20 MINS, PLUS CHILLING | **COOK TIME** 30 MINS

CRÈME BRÛLÉE

CRÈME BRÛLÉE TO THE FRENCH, CREMA CATALANA TO THE SPANISH, THIS VANILLA CUSTARD DESSERT IS RICH, CREAMY AND AN INDULGENT TREAT

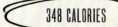

348 CALORIES

INGREDIENTS

- 75ML | 2.5FLOZ KAHLÚA (COFFEE LIQUEUR)
- 30ML | 1FLOZ STRONG COFFEE GRANULES
- 100G | 3.5OZ CASTER SUGAR
- 300ML | 10.1FLOZ DOUBLE/HEAVY CREAM
- 200ML | 6.8FLOZ FULL-FAT/WHOLE MILK
- 6 MEDIUM EGG YOLKS
- 2TSP CORNFLOUR/CORNSTARCH

FOR THE TOPPING:
- 30G | 1.1OZ CASTER SUGAR

YOU WILL NEED:
- 8X 100ML | 3.4FLOZ RAMEKINS

STEP 1 Reserve 1tbsp Kahlúa and put the remaining 60ml | 2floz in a pan with the coffee granules and 30g | 1.1oz caster sugar. Bring to the boil and simmer for 5-8 mins until thick and syrupy, then stir in the reserved Kahlúa. Pour into a small bowl or jug and wipe the pan clean.

STEP 2 Gently warm the cream and milk in a pan until steaming, but not boiling. Meanwhile, heat the oven to 150°C (130°C fan) | 300°F | gas 2. Whisk the remaining 70g | 2.5oz caster sugar with the egg yolks and cornflour until thick and creamy.

STEP 3 Once the cream mixture is steaming, carefully pour it over the whisked egg yolks in a steady stream, stirring continuously. Mix in the cooled syrup.

STEP 4 Strain the mixture through a fine sieve into a large jug. If the consistency is foamy, leave for a few mins to settle, then use a spoon to remove the rest.

STEP 5 Put the ramekins in a large, deep roasting tin, then divide the custard between them. Pour a kettleful of just boiled water into the tin so that it reaches halfway up the ramekins. Bake for 30 mins until the custard is just set with a slight wobble.

STEP 6 Remove the ramekins from the water and cool on a wire rack, then cover and chill for at least 2 hrs, or overnight.

STEP 7 When ready to serve, sprinkle over the caster sugar and tap off any excess. For best results, use a blowtorch to gently caramelise the tops, or put under a hot grill until melted. Put aside for 1-2 mins until the top has set before serving.

DESSERTS

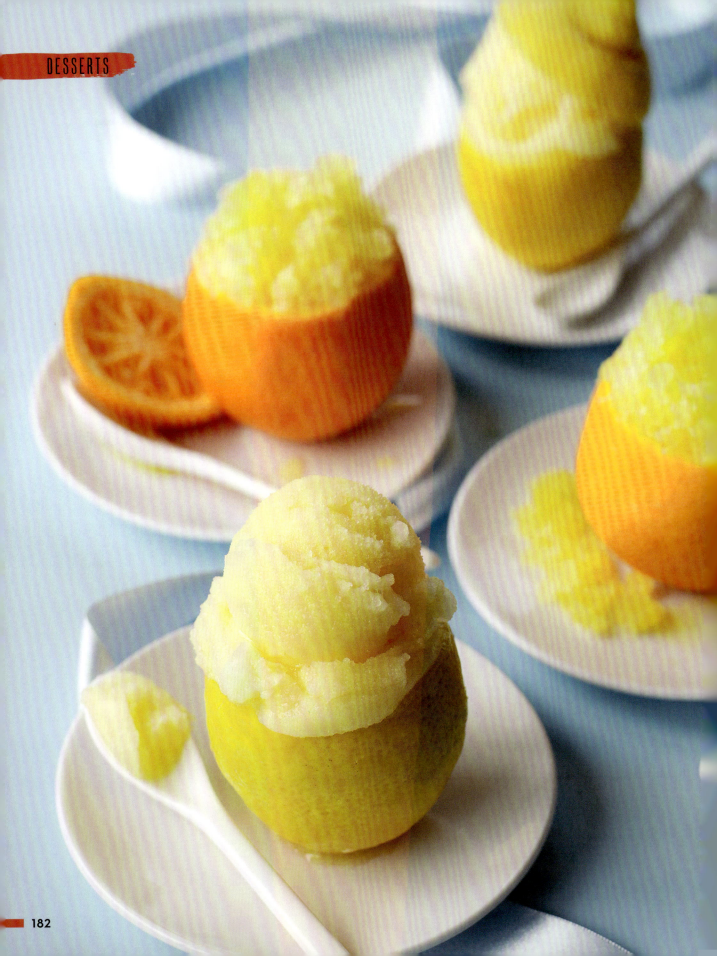

182

SERVINGS 6   **PREP TIME 20 MINS, PLUS FREEZING**   **COOK TIME 5 MINS**

LEMON SORBET

THIS REFRESHING SORBETTE AL LIMONE WILL NOT ONLY TRANSPORT YOU TO YOUR HOLIDAYS ON THE MED, BUT IT'S FAT-FREE TOO

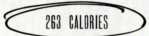

263 CALORIES

INGREDIENTS

JUICE OF 6 UNWAXED LEMONS, PLUS THE GRATED ZEST OF 3
350G | 12.3OZ CASTER SUGAR
PULP OF 3 PASSION FRUIT

YOU WILL NEED:
900ML | 30.4FLOZ RIGID CONTAINER, SUITABLE FOR FREEZING
ICE-CREAM MACHINE

STEP 1 Put the lemon zest and juice in a pan with the sugar and 200ml | 6.8floz water. Simmer gently for 5 mins. Remove from the heat, stir in the passion-fruit pulp and set aside for 10 mins to cool.

STEP 2 Strain the mixture into a measuring jug, pressing with a spoon to get as much through as possible. Top up to 750ml | 25.4floz with cold water. Pour into an ice-cream machine and churn to make a spoonable mixture with fine crystals. Transfer to rigid container and freeze.

STEP 3 Transfer to the fridge at least 20 mins before serving. Serve in hollowed-out lemons and oranges, if liked, or glasses.

DESSERTS

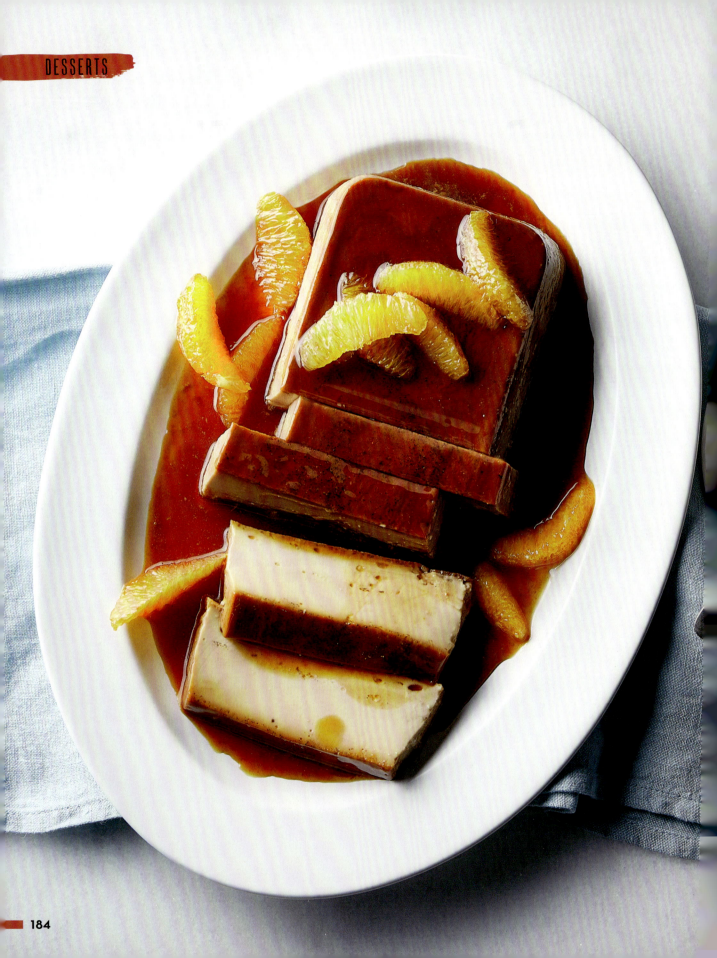

SERVINGS 8 | **PREP TIME 20 MINS, PLUS AT LEAST 4 HRS CHILLING** | **COOK TIME 1 HR 20 MINS**

CRÈME CARAMEL

ESPRESSO AND VANILLA COMBINE PERFECTLY IN THIS RICH AND CREAMY FRENCH CLASSIC, ALSO KNOWN AS FLAN IN SPAIN

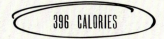
396 CALORIES

INGREDIENTS

- 150G | 5.3OZ CASTER SUGAR
- 3 MEDIUM EGGS, PLUS 3 YOLKS
- 120G | 4.2OZ SOFT LIGHT BROWN SUGAR
- 1 VANILLA POD, HALVED, SEEDS SCRAPED
- 300ML | 10.1FLOZ DOUBLE/HEAVY CREAM
- 300ML | 10.1FLOZ FULL-FAT WHOLE MILK
- 1TBSP ESPRESSO INSTANT COFFEE POWDER
- 50ML | 1.7FLOZ KAHLÚA LIQUEUR (OPTIONAL)
- 2 LARGE ORANGES, SEGMENTED, TO SERVE (OPTIONAL)

YOU WILL NEED:
1.2-L (2.5-PT) CAPACITY LOAF TIN, LIGHTLY OILED

STEP 1 Heat the oven to 150°C (130°C fan) | 300°F | gas 2. Put the caster sugar and 60ml | 2floz water in a saucepan and stir over a medium heat until the sugar dissolves. Increase the heat to high and boil for 8-10 mins until the sugar turns a dark caramel colour. Carefully pour into the loaf tin and tilt to coat the bottom and sides. Put in a deep-sided roasting tin and set aside.

STEP 2 Whisk together the eggs, egg yolks and brown sugar in a large bowl.

STEP 3 Put the remaining ingredients, except the oranges, in a large saucepan. Bring to a simmer, then remove from the heat and whisk into the egg mixture.

STEP 4 Strain the custard through a sieve, discarding the vanilla pod, then pour into the loaf tin. Add boiling water to the roasting tin to come two-thirds up the sides of the loaf tin, then bake for 1 hr 20 mins until set around the edges, with a wobble in the middle. Set aside to cool, then cover and chill for at least 4 hrs or, ideally, overnight.

STEP 5 Run a knife around the edge of the tin to loosen, then invert onto a plate. Slice and serve with orange segments, if liked.

DESSERTS

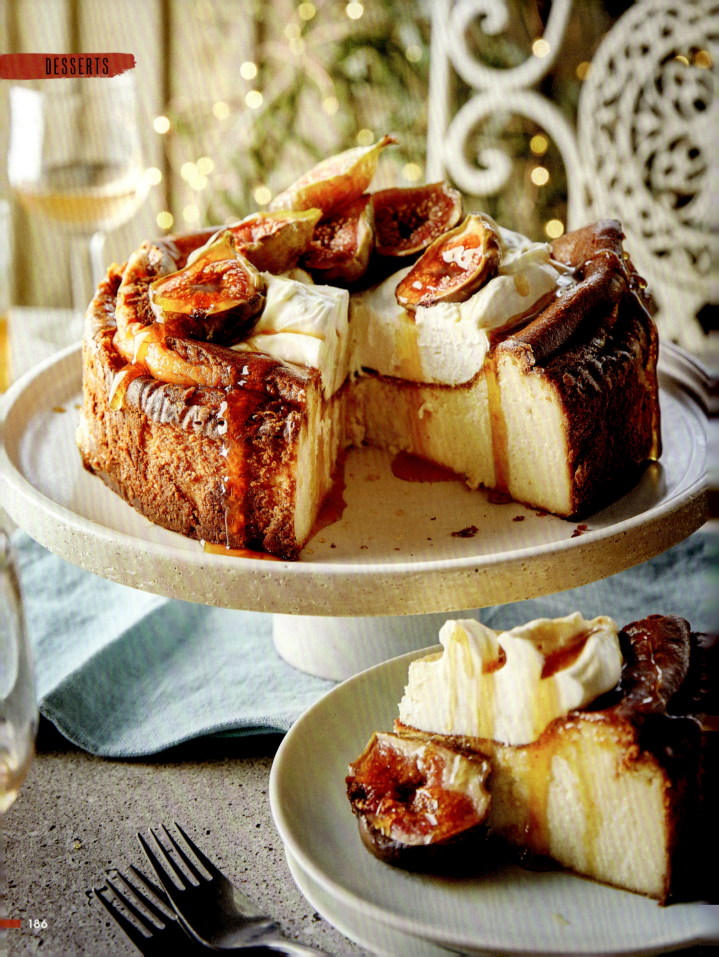

SERVINGS 12 | **PREP TIME 30 MINS, PLUS OVERNIGHT CHILLING** | **COOK TIME 1 HR 40 MINS**

BASQUE-STYLE BURNT CHEESECAKE WITH HONEY ROASTED FIGS

THIS RUSTIC SPANISH BEAUTY IS THE EASIEST CHEESECAKE YOU'LL EVER MAKE. DON'T BE PUT OFF BY THE DEEPLY CARAMELISED EXTERIOR – IT IS THE SECRET TO THIS DESSERT'S CARAMEL FLAVOUR

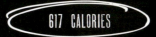

617 CALORIES

INGREDIENTS

- 840G | 29.6OZ PHILADELPHIA CREAM CHEESE
- 325G | 11.5OZ CASTER SUGAR
- 4 MEDIUM EGGS, PLUS 2 YOLKS, BEATEN
- 600ML | 20.3FLOZ DOUBLE/HEAVY CREAM
- 1 TBSP VANILLA BEAN PASTE
- 5 TBSP PLAIN FLOUR
- 6-8 FRESH FIGS, HALVED
- 1 ROSEMARY SPRIG
- 4 TBSP RUNNY HONEY
- 4 TBSP SWEET SHERRY

YOU WILL NEED:
20CM | 7.9" LOOSE-BOTTOM CAKE TIN, THE BASE AND SIDES LINED WITH BAKING PAPER, EXTENDING 3-4CM | 1.2-1.6" ABOVE THE RIM

STEP 1 Heat the oven to 160°C (140°C fan) | 325°F | gas 3. In a large bowl, use an electric mixer on low speed to beat the Philadelphia and sugar together. Add the eggs and yolks, one at a time, followed by 400g | 14.1oz of the cream and the vanilla bean paste, mixing until smooth. Finally, mix in the flour.

STEP 2 Pour the mixture into the prepared tin then bake for 1 hr 40 mins. The top should be a deep golden colour and the centre will still have a good wiggle. Cool in the tin, then cover and chill overnight.

STEP 3 For the figs, heat the oven to 220°C (200°C fan) | 425°F | gas 7. Put the figs in a roasting tin, cut side up. Add the rosemary, and drizzle over the honey and sherry. Roast for 15 mins until the figs have darkened in colour and the syrup is thickened.

STEP 4 When ready to serve, remove the cheesecake from the tin and transfer to a serving plate. Whip the remaining cream to soft peaks then dollop on top of the cheesecake. Top with the figs and drizzle over the honey syrup.

DESSERTS

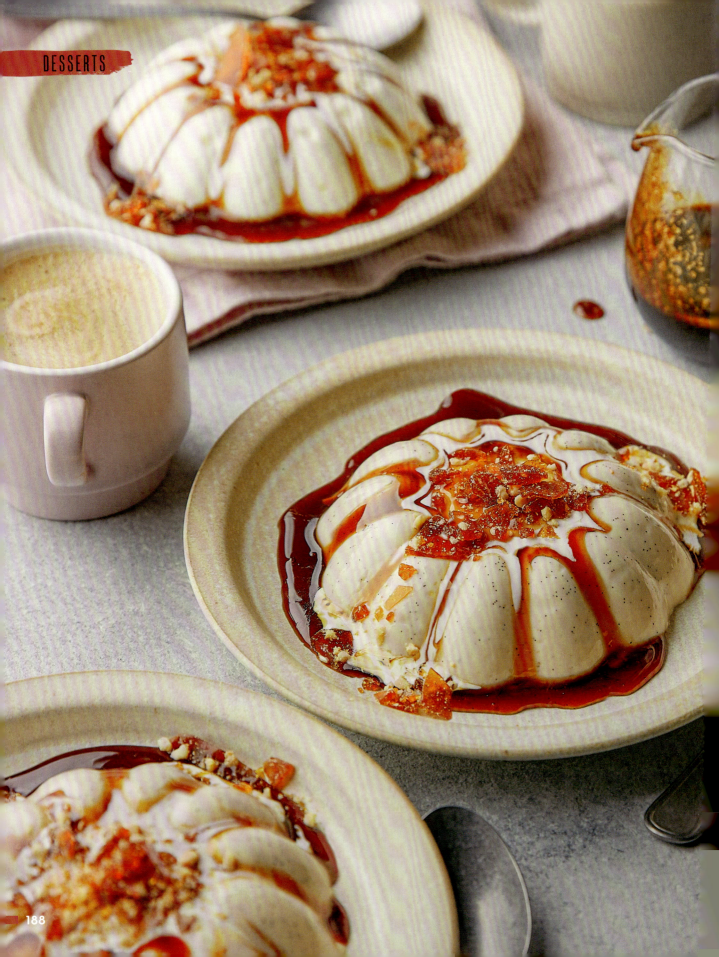

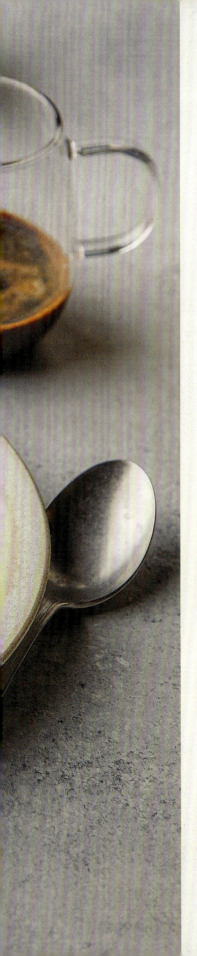

SERVINGS 6 | **PREP TIME 10 MINS, PLUS SETTING** | **COOK TIME 5 MINS**

LATTE PANNA COTTA

SWEET AND LIGHT, THIS ITALIAN PANNA COTTA'S COFFEE AND HAZELNUT SYRUP GIVES A SOPHISTICATED HIT

196 CALORIES

INGREDIENTS

3 GELATINE LEAVES
500ML | 16.9FLOZ WHOLE MILK
100ML | 3.4FLOZ SINGLE/LIGHT CREAM, PLUS EXTRA FOR DRIZZLING
1 VANILLA POD, SPLIT LENGTHWAYS, SEEDS SCRAPED
50G | 1.8OZ CASTER SUGAR
2TSP HAZELNUT LIQUEUR (OPTIONAL)

FOR THE SYRUP:
100G | 3.5OZ CASTER SUGAR
150ML | 5FLOZ STRONG ESPRESSO COFFEE
1TBSP HAZELNUT LIQUEUR (OPTIONAL)
PRALINE, TO SERVE (OPTIONAL)

YOU WILL NEED:
6X 120ML | 4FLOZ DARIOLE MOULDS, LIGHTLY GREASED

STEP 1 Soften the gelatine in cold water for 5 mins. Put the milk, cream, vanilla pod and seeds in a saucepan and warm over a low heat until steaming. Stir in the sugar to dissolve and the hazelnut liqueur, if using.

STEP 2 Squeeze the softened gelatine to remove excess water, then whisk into the milk mixture, making sure it's fully dissolved. Strain; discard the vanilla pod. Divide the mixture between the moulds and chill for at least 4 hrs or overnight.

STEP 3 For the syrup, put the sugar and coffee in a small pan and simmer to reduce by half. Add the liqueur, if using; leave to cool.

STEP 4 To serve, briefly dip the moulds in hot water to release the panna cottas, then invert onto plates. Pour over 2tbsp syrup and serve with some praline, if liked.

DESSERTS

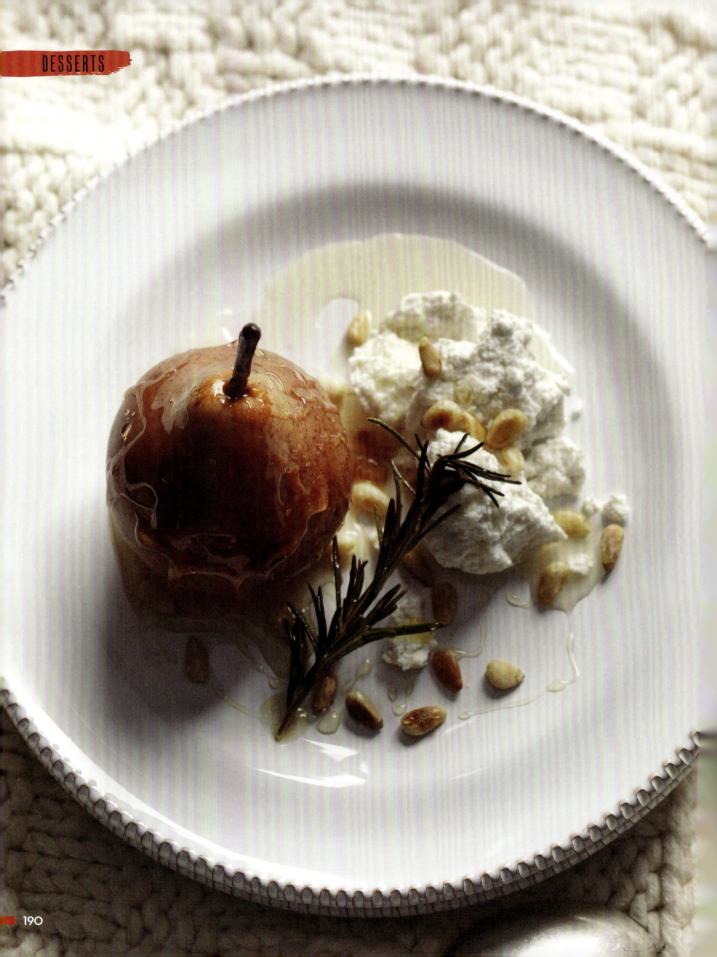

SERVINGS 4   PREP TIME 10 MINS, PLUS SETTING   COOK TIME 35 MINS

POACHED PEARS WITH FRESH RICOTTA, HONEY AND PINE NUTS

THIS MEDITERRANEAN DESSERT MAY BE LESS CALORIFIC THAN MANY, BUT IT'S JUST AS DELICIOUS AND WONDERFULLY AROMATIC FROM THE FRESH ROSEMARY

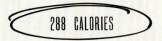

288 CALORIES

INGREDIENTS

4 JUST-RIPE PEARS
2TBSP HONEY
2TBSP BUTTER
4 ROSEMARY SPRIGS
A SQUEEZE OF LEMON JUICE
100G | 3.5OZ RICOTTA CHEESE, WHIPPED UNTIL CREAMY
2TBSP PINE NUTS, TOASTED IN A DRY PAN
2TBSP HONEY AND ROSEMARY, TO SERVE

STEP 1 Pre-heat the oven to 180°C (160°C fan) | 350°F | gas 4. Core the pears and cut a horizontal sliver from the bases, then stand them upright in a dish small enough to fit them snugly.

STEP 2 Drizzle with honey, dot with butter, then tuck the rosemary sprigs in and around them. Add a squeeze of lemon juice and a splash of water. Cover with foil and bake for about 35 mins until the pears are soft, but are still holding their shape.

STEP 3 Serve with juices from the dish, spoonfuls of ricotta, a scattering of toasted pine nuts, a drizzle of honey and a rosemary sprig, if preferred.

DESSERTS

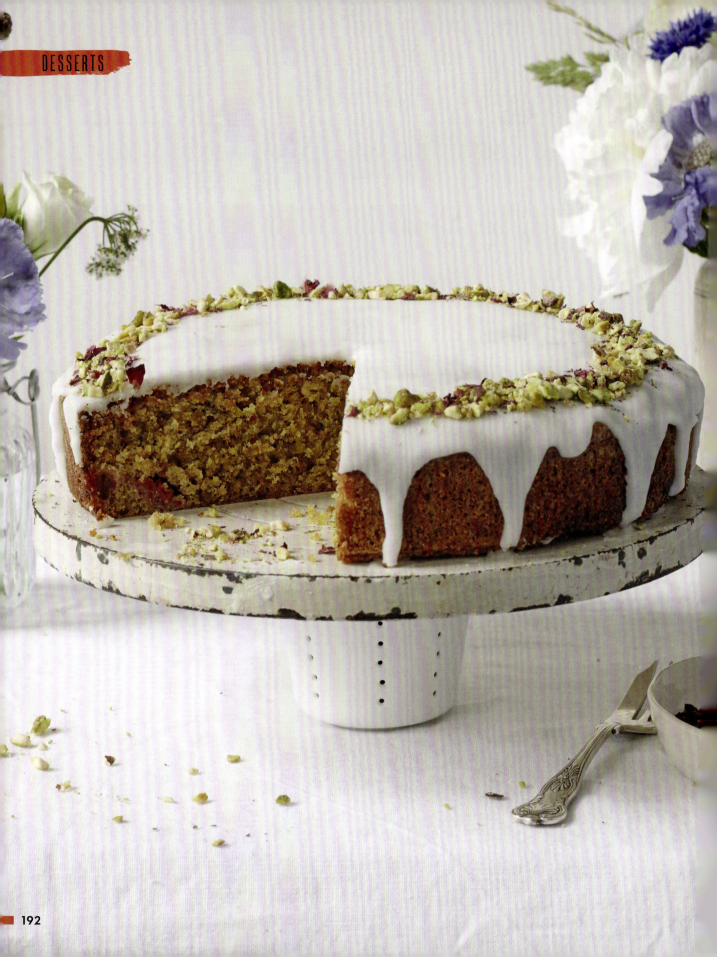

PISTACHIO, ROSE AND OLIVE OIL CAKE

SERVINGS 10-12 | PREP TIME 20 MINS, PLUS SETTING | COOK TIME 1 HR

THE POPULAR MEDITERRANEAN OLIVE OIL CAKE GETS A PERSIAN MAKEOVER

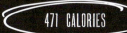

471 CALORIES

INGREDIENTS

- 200G | 7OZ PISTACHIO KERNELS
- 200ML | 6.8FLOZ LIGHT OLIVE OIL
- 250G | 8.8OZ GOLDEN CASTER SUGAR
- 1/2TSP ROSEWATER
- 4 LARGE EGGS
- 125G | 4.4OZ PLAIN FLOUR
- 1 1/2TSP BAKING POWDER
- 150G | 5.3OZ RASPBERRIES, HALVED

FOR THE ICING:
- 200G | 7OZ ICING SUGAR
- DRIED ROSE PETALS, TO DECORATE

YOU WILL NEED:
- 23CM | 9IN SPRINGFORM TIN, GREASED AND LINED

STEP 1 Heat the oven to 180°C (160°C fan) | 350°F | gas 4. Blitz the pistachios in a food processor until finely ground, setting aside 2tbsp to decorate. In a stand mixer or with a hand-held electric mixer, beat the oil with the sugar, rosewater and eggs until pale and fluffy, then fold through the pistachios, flour and baking powder until well combined. Carefully fold through the raspberries.

STEP 2 Transfer to the cake tin and bake for 55 mins–1hr, until a skewer inserted in the centre comes out clean. Leave to cool in the cake tin.

STEP 3 Once cooled, sift the icing sugar into a bowl to remove any lumps. Gradually add 3-4tbsp water until it's a smooth but spreadable consistency. Spread over the top of the cake, allowing it to drip slightly over the edges. Leave this to firm up slightly then decorate with the reserved pistachios and roses by creating a ring around the edge of the cake.

DESSERTS

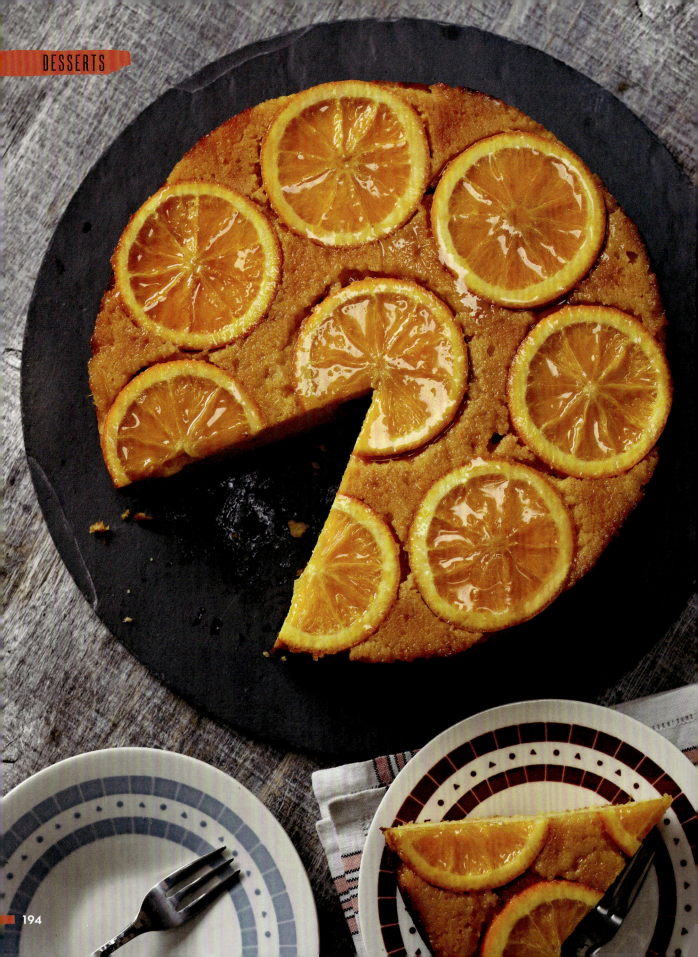

SERVINGS 10 | **PREP TIME 30 MINS, PLUS COOLING** | **COOK TIME 45 MINS**

ORANGE POLENTA CAKE

THIS ITALIAN CAKE CONTAINS AN INGREDIENT YOU WOULDN'T NORMALLY EXPECT TO FIND IN A DESSERT, BUT TRUST US – IT WORKS A TREAT

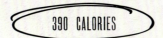

390 CALORIES

INGREDIENTS

- 65G | 2.3OZ GOLDEN CASTER SUGAR
- 5 ORANGES – ZEST 2, THEN SLICE, PLUS JUICE FROM 3
- 150G | 5.3OZ UNSALTED BUTTER, SOFTENED
- 200G | 7OZ GROUND ALMONDS
- 50G | 1.8OZ GLUTEN-FREE FLOUR, SIFTED
- 50G | 1.8OZ FINE POLENTA
- 1½TSP GLUTEN-FREE BAKING POWDER
- 2TBSP HONEY
- 4 LARGE EGGS, LIGHTLY BEATEN
- 300G | 10.6OZ SWEET POTATOES, MASHED AND COOLED

YOU WILL NEED:
22CM (8.7IN) LOOSE-BASED CAKE TIN, GREASED AND LINED WITH BAKING PAPER

STEP 1 Heat oven to 180°C (160°C fan) | 350°F | gas 4. In a small pan, heat 50g | 1.8oz of the sugar, adding the orange zest and juice. Bubble until syrupy, then pour half onto the base of the prepared tin. Cube 25g | 0.9oz of the butter and dot over the syrup, then add a layer of orange slices.

STEP 2 Mix the almonds with the flour, polenta and baking powder.

STEP 3 In a separate bowl, cream the remaining butter with remaining sugar and honey until smooth. Gradually beat eggs into butter mix, adding a little of the dry ingredient mix now and again to prevent curdling. Fold in rest of almond mix and sweet potato. Spoon into the tin and bake for 35-45 mins.

STEP 4 Cool in the tin for 5 mins before tipping the cake out on to a wire rack to cool. Once cool, pierce with a skewer before pouring over the rest of the syrup.

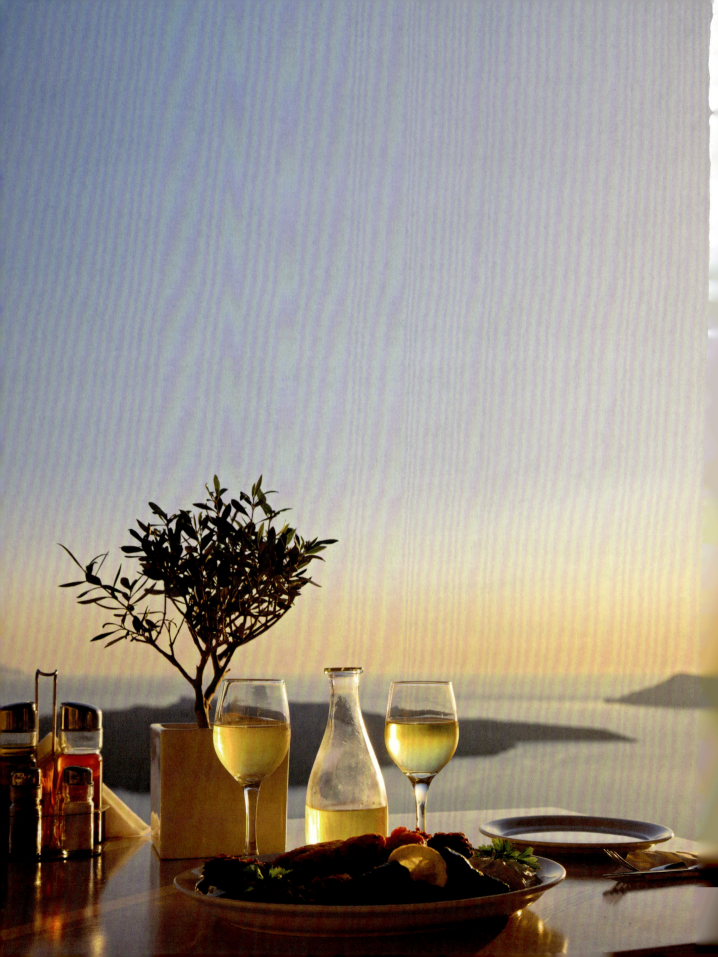

The *Mediterranean* DIET BOOK

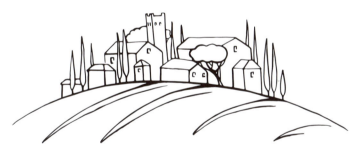

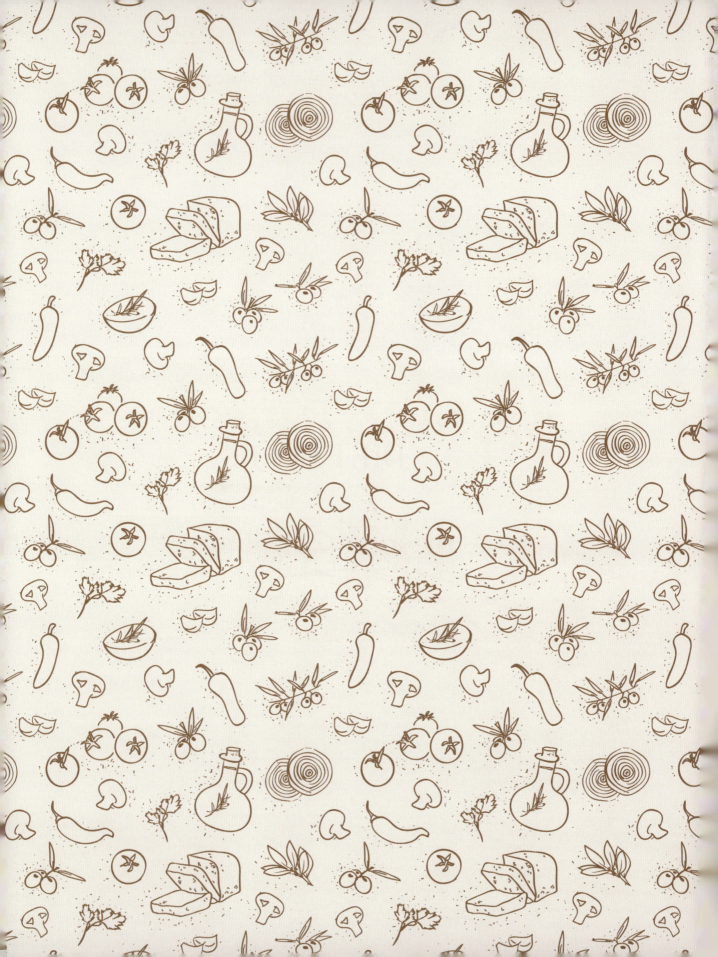